Jennifer Perillo is a food writer and recipe deve
who runs the blog In Jennie's Kitchen, whic
been featured in *Food 52, Saveur, Fine Coc
Serious Eats, Bon Appetit*, and Oprah.com. Sl
worked as the Consulting Food Editor at Wo
Mother magazine, and contributed to a variety ог
print and online publications and food websites,
including Food Network, Relish, Food 52, Cuisinart,
Parade, and Parenting. She is the author of *Homemade with Love*.

www.injennieskitchen.com

 @ JenniferPerillo

 Facebook.com/injennieskitchen

THE BEGINNER'S GUIDE TO INTERMITTENT KETO

First published in Great Britain in 2019 by

Quercus Editions Ltd
Carmelite House
50 Victoria Embankment
London EC4Y 0DZ

An Hachette UK company

A CIP catalogue record for this book is available
from the British Library.

ISBN 978 1 52940 119 6

10 9 8 7 6 5 4 3 2 1

Typeset by CC Production

Printed and bound in Great Britain by Clays Ltd, Elcograf S.p.A.

THE BEGINNER'S GUIDE TO
INTERMITTENT KETO

JENNIFER PERILLO

Quercus

Contents

Part I
Introduction to Intermittent Fasting and the Keto Diet

Part II
Meal Plans and Recipes

BREAKFAST

LUNCH

DINNER

TREATS & BEVERAGES

BASICS

Part III
Resources

Part I

Introduction to Intermittent Fasting and the Keto Diet

We are what we eat. Sounds like a simple, straightforward statement, right? Let's take it one step further, though, and consider *how* we eat. Chances are you're looking to make a change if you're reading this book. Maybe the goal is weight loss, trying to lose those last stubborn ten pounds. Perhaps you're exploring changing your diet for preventive measures to put yourself on a better health track for the future.

Intermittent fasting and ketosis, also referred to as IF and keto, are probably familiar, or at least recognizable, terms since you bought this book in the first place. Unlike fad diets, where you might see fast results but are hard to maintain long term, both intermittent fasting and keto target the root systems of how you consume food, and the choices you make with each meal. Implemented properly, intermittent fasting and keto are lifestyle changes,

and long-term solutions for a healthier, happier you.

Today's availability of information means everything we want to know about anything is at our fingertips, or with a swipe of one. That same convenience can often leave you with an overload of information. How do you decipher it all, and determine if intermittent fasting and keto are right for you? That's the goal of this book. I did a deep dive into both lifestyles, and analyzed the benefits of both practices, implemented on their own, and combined, so you can cut straight to the chase, and get started on your Intermittent Keto journey.

Before you set out making changes, approach this as you would any recipe—read the directions from beginning to end first. Make sure you understand not just how to do intermittent fasting and cook keto-friendly meals, but the science behind it all. Reading all the introductory material will make the transition to this new lifestyle easier and give you a foundation to see the 4-week Plan through to completion. Tempting as it might be to skip straight to the 4-week Plan and the recipes, keep in mind a solid foundation is the key to success. The words between this introduction and the recipes provide the bricks and mortar to build a solid start.

Be prepared for the naysayers. We'll talk about this more in the Before You Get Started section on page 21. Everyone is an expert nowadays, ready to share their opinions whether welcome or not. Remember only YOU are the expert on you. Once you've read through the following sections, you'll know if Intermittent Keto is right for you. Of course, if you have any underlying health concerns, always consult your doctor or medical practitioner before making any changes to your diet and lifestyle.

What is Ketosis?

On the surface, carbs are a quick, often fast and inexpensive form of nutrition to power you through each day. Think about all those grab-n-go snacks we associate with breakfast—granola bars, fruit-filled smoothies, muffins. We start our mornings with carbohydrates, and keep piling them on as the day progresses.

Just because something works doesn't mean it's the most efficient means. The tissues and cells that make up our bodies need energy to perform everyday functions to keep us alive. There are two primary sources from which they can draw energy. One source is carbohydrates, which convert to glucose. That is the current model most of us follow. There's an alternative fuel, though, and a surprising one: fat. Yes, the very thing you've been told to limit eating your entire life might just be the resource you need to jumpstart your metabolism. Organic compounds, called ketones, are released when our bodies metabolize food and break down fatty acids. Ketones can be used for energy to keep our cells and muscles functioning.

You've likely heard the word metabolism throughout your life, but what does it mean exactly? At its root, the term simply refers to the chemical reactions required in any living organism to stay alive. Of course, metabolism is anything but simple given the complexities of the human body. Our bodies are constantly at work. Even when we're sleeping, our cells are always building and repairing. They need a never-ending supply of energy.

Glucose, which is what carbs break down into once we eat them, is one way to fuel our metabolism. Our current nutrition guidelines focus on carbs as the primary source of energy. Factor in any additional sugars we eat, and the recommended daily servings of fruit, starchy vegetables, grains, and plant-based forms of protein (i.e. beans), there's no lack of glucose in our bodies. The problem with this model of energy consumption is it leaves our body like a hamster running on a wheel. We're burning energy but getting nowhere when it comes to output, especially if we're consuming more carbs than our body can use in a day's work.

There's the other form of energy I mentioned: fat. How does that work exactly? Is it possible tapping into that alternative fuel source will help our bodies burn energy more efficiently, with greater overall benefit to our health? We're back to that old idea of you are what you eat, except now think about the principal theory as *you burn what you eat*. That's where ketosis comes into play. Switching to a high-fat, moderate-protein, low-carb diet, allows your body to enter into a state of ketosis, wherein you metabolize fat, triggering a release of ketones to fuel the functions of our elaborate inner workings. The liver releases ketones after fatty acids are broken down.

Achieving a state of ketosis is about balance, but not the kind you're used to when it comes to eating. It turns out our current food pyramid is upside down. Instead of consuming an inordinate amount of carbohydrates for energy, a more efficient plan for fueling your body focuses fats at the top, making up 60 to 80% of your diet, protein in the middle at 20 to 30%, and carbs (really glucose in disguise) way at the bottom, just 5 to 10% of your daily eating plan.

Keto vs. Paleo

Evolution offers us many benefits. The ability to use fire and electricity to cook our food is proof alone that progress can be a good thing. Somewhere between our hunter-gatherer foraging lifestyle and today's modern world, a big disconnect happened. Sure, we have longer lifespans, but what about the quality of those extra years from a health perspective? The sluggish feeling that never seems to go away may not be just because you need to get extra sleep (though sleep is always a good thing!).

If food is fuel for our bodies, then it's safe to say that what we eat impacts our productivity. Put diesel in a car designed to run on gasoline, and the effects are disastrous. Is it possible our bodies are in a similar state today, the result of our systems having evolved to rely on carbs for energy as food availability became more consistent, instead of fat from our early days of existence. I realize this sounds an awful lot like advocating for a paleo diet, but while the ketogenic lifestyle looks similar, the underlying principle to Keto is vastly different. Keto is about creating a synergy between what you eat and the way your body functions—that's why the focus is on a specific manipulation of macronutrients (fat, protein, carbohydrates, fiber, and fluids). Every calorie is made up of a specific macronutrient. Understanding why you're making such specific food choices is key to comprehending the bigger picture.

Fiber, for example, keeps us "regular" because it helps food pass through the digestive system. What goes in must come out. Fiber is essential to that process. Protein aids in tissue repair, producing enzymes, building bones, muscle, and skin. Fluids keep us hydrated, akin to watering a garden—without it, our cells, tissues, and organs cannot function properly.

Carbohydrate's primary role is to provide energy; however, to do so, the body converts it into glucose, which has a ripple effect throughout the rest of your body. Carb consumption is a delicate balance for people with diabetes because of its relationship to insulin production from increased blood sugar levels. Healthy fats support cell growth, protect our organs, help keep us warm, and have the ability to provide energy, but only when carbohydrates are consumed in limited quantities. I'll explain more about why and how that happens shortly.

Carbs vs. Net Carbs

Carbohydrates exist in some form in almost every food source. Total elimination is impossible, and not practical. We do need some to function. It's important to know this to understand the reason why some foods fall into the restricted category on a Keto diet, but also why some of those choices are better than others.

Fiber counts as a carb in the nutritional breakdown of a meal. What's important to note is that fiber does not significantly affect your blood sugar, a good thing since it's an essential macronutrient that helps us digest food properly. By subtracting the amount of fiber from the amount of carbs in the nutritional tally of an ingredient or finished recipe, you're left with what's called "net carbs".

Think about your paycheck before taxes (gross), and after (net). A terrible analogy, perhaps, since no one enjoys paying taxes, but an effective one in trying to understand carbs vs. net carbs and how to track them. You put a certain amount of carbs into your body, but not all of them affect your blood sugar level.

This doesn't mean you can go crazy with wholegrain pasta because it is high in fibre. Even though it's a better choice than white flour pasta, overall you should be limiting net carbs to 20 to 25 grams per day. To put that in perspective, two ounces of uncooked wholegrain pasta has about 35 grams of carbohydrates and only 7 grams of total fiber. Pasta and bread are probably two of the main things about which people will ask "but don't you miss them?" The best way to answer them is by sharing all the things you can eat (see the Keto Cheat Sheet on page 37).

How Long Does It Take For Ketosis To Kick In?

The short answer is most people transition into ketosis within 1 to 3 days. It can take some people a full week for that to happen, as all bodies are different. Factors that affect how quickly you enter ketosis include your current body weight, diet, and activity level.

In order to enter ketosis your body needs to first

burn through its glycogen (glucose) supply. Once glycogen is depleted, your body signals it's time to start breaking down those fatty acids as an alternative source of energy. Over the next few days, the liver gets the message to begin excreting ketones. This last part of the process signals you're in ketosis. The early stage is a mild ketosis, as ketone levels will be relatively low until you maintain ketosis for a steady period of time. You can measure ketone levels formally (see page 23), but you might start to notice some physiological changes that show you're in ketosis, such as Keto Flu or Keto Breath. They are not as severe or dramatic as they sound, and the benefits of ketosis might outweigh the phase-in period for your defined goals, but it's good to familiarize yourself with the symptoms nonetheless (see pages 27 and 30).

Intermittent Fasting: What Does It Mean?

S ay the phrase, "today I will fast" to yourself, and think about the first thing that comes to mind. Let me guess, was it "I don't want to starve"? You're not alone in this common misconception, so let's break it down, and make it easier to digest (pun very much intended!).

Fasting vs. Starvation

Fasting is a conscious choice. What sets fasting apart from starvation is that it's a decision you make to intentionally not eat. The length of time you choose to do it, and the purpose, be it for religious reasons, weight loss, or a detox, is not something forced upon you. Fasting is done at will. Done properly, fasting can also have positive effects on our overall health.

Starvation is brought upon unwilling people by a set of circumstances out of their control. Famine, poverty, war being just a few reasons for such a catastrophic situation. Starvation is a severe deficiency in calories that can lead to organ damage, and eventually death. No one chooses to starve.

Once I thought about it from this perspective it made perfect sense, and it was so much easier to wrap my head around the idea. Yes, I was skeptical about fasting at first, too. Before acknowledging the difference between the two, my first reaction was always "why would anyone choose to starve themselves?" The reality is, anyone who decides to fast is only choosing not to eat for a predetermined period of time. Even peaceful protests that use fasting as a means to an end have a defined goal for fasting.

Will you feel hungry while fasting?

To answer that, let's put the question in perspective. The truth is we all fast once a day. We often eat our last meal a few hours before going to sleep, and with the exception of nursing newborns, I can't think of anyone who eats the moment they wake. Even if you only average six hours of sleep a night, it's likely you're already fasting 10 hours a day. Now let's add the idea of intermittent to the mix. Intermittent means something that is not continuous. When applying that to the idea of fasting, it means you're elongating the amount of time before you eat after your last meal (the word breakfast when broken down means just that, breaking the fast).

Since our bodies are already accustomed to fasting once a day, the bigger issue is mind over matter. Let's get back to the question of will you feel hungry. The first week may be an adjustment as you get used to the extended the period of time of your new fasting goal. The 4-week Plan on page 53 builds the fasting part of your day onto your sleeping hours, to help with this adjustment. It's quite possible your body will start to feel hungry around whatever time you're currently used to eating breakfast if it's before noon, but that will adjust within a few days.

In anticipation of the change you're about to make, try pushing back your first meal of the day by 30 minutes every day for a week before starting the 4-week Plan. This way when you begin the schedule laid out on page 50 you'll just need to adjust your timing for your final meal of the day once you begin week two of the plan for the noon to 6pm eating schedule.

Why Choose Intermittent Fasting?

Now that we've cleared up what it really means to fast, and you realize it's a conscious choice to not eat for a period of time, you might be still be wondering "but why bother?" The main reason intermittent fasting (commonly referred to as IF) has taken the diet world by storm is its ability to promote weight loss. Metabolism is often categorized as one function of the human body. In reality, metabolism involves two essential reactions: catabolism and anabolism.

Catabolism is the part of metabolism wherein our bodies break down the food we consume. During catabolism, complex molecules are broken down into smaller units, releasing energy. Anabolism then uses that energy to begin the process of rebuilding and repairing our bodies, growing new cells, and maintaining tissues. Technically speaking, catabolism and anabolism happen simultaneously, but the rate at which they occur is different. A traditional eating schedule, where we spend the majority of our day eating, means our bodies have less time to spend in the second phase of metabolism: anabolism. A little confusing, perhaps, because the processes are interdependent, but remember the rates at which they occur differ. The important takeaway here is that fasting for an elongated period allows for maximum efficiency in the metabolic processes.

Another amazing side effect of fasting, even for an intermittent period as outlined in this book, is a resurgence in mental acuity. Numerous studies show that contrary to popular thought, fasting makes you more aware and focused, not tired or light-headed as one might assume. Many point to evolution and our ability to survive as a species. Long before food preservation was possible, mental awareness was necessary at all times to live from day to day, regardless of how plentiful food resources may have been.

Scientific research points towards neurogenesis kicking into high gear during periods of fasting. Neurogenesis is the growth and development of nerve tissue in the brain.

All roads lead towards one exceptionally important conclusion when it comes to fasting: it allows your body time to do more of the "behind the scenes" work necessary. The longer you extend the window between eating your last meal of one day and consuming the first meal of the following one, the more time your body has to focus on cellular regeneration and tissue repair at all levels.

Are Liquids Allowed When Fasting?

There's one last important detail to note about intermittent fasting. Unlike religious fasting, which generally restricts consuming any food or liquids during the fast period, IF allows you to consume certain liquids. Technically speaking, the moment you consume anything with calories a fast is broken. Looking at it through the lens of using intermittent fasting for its weight-loss benefits means we can apply different rules, so to speak.

Bone broth (recipe on page 127) is recommended to replenish vitamins, minerals, and maintain sodium levels. Coffee and tea are allowed, preferably without any added milk or cream, and absolutely no sweeteners. There are two schools of thought on adding fat to your coffee or tea. Provided it's only a high-fat addition such as coconut oil and butter to make bulletproof coffee (see the recipe on page 122), many Keto advocates think it's fine since it doesn't disrupt ketosis. Adding MCT oil is believed to boost energy levels and keep you feeling satiated, as well. Purists adhere to plain coffee or tea. You should do what works best for you, provided it doesn't kick you out of ketosis (there are ways to test for this, see page 23).

Let's not forget water, as staying well hydrated is essential to any healthy lifestyle choices. Caffeine can be especially depleting, so make sure to balance coffee consumption with water intake, too.

The Power of Intermittent Fasting & Keto Combined

By now, the benefits of intermittent fasting and adhering to a Keto diet should be evident. What you might not have pieced together is the connection between the two. When you're in ketosis, that process of breaking down fatty acids to produce ketones for fuel is actually what the body does to keep itself going when you're fasting. What does it mean to combine the two, and why bother blending these lifestyles and ways of eating?

Fasting for 1 to 2 days has a significant effect when eating a traditional carb-centric diet. After the initial phase of burning glucose (i.e. carbohydrates) for energy, your body naturally switches over to burning fat for fuel.

You see where I'm going here, right? If it takes 24 to 48 hours for your body to switch over to burning fat for fuel, imagine the effects of combining inter-mittent fasting with Keto. Maintaining a constant state of ketosis means your body is already burning fat for fuel. This means the longer you spend in a state of fasting, you're burning fat longer. Inter-mittent fasting combined with Keto makes fasting's weight-loss effects more efficient, often resulting in more weight loss than traditional diets. The pro-longed time between your last and first meals of the day means extra fat-burning capabilities for your body.

Ketosis is often used in body building because it's a safe way to shed fat without losing muscle. Weight loss is only good when it's the right weight, and we all need our muscle mass to stay healthy.

How Does It Work?

Switching to the Keto diet is a huge lifestyle change. For that reason, it's best to ease into the intermittent fasting aspect of this program. Let your body adjust to a new way of eating, adapt to burning fat for fuel, and deal with any possible side effects (remember Keto flu is a possibility), before incorporating inter-mittent fasting into your eating routine, or in this case extending the period of not eating. That's why you'll notice intermittent fasting is introduced in Week Two of the 4-week Plan.

During the phase-in period, you'll want to take

note of eating times. Even before you incorporate the intermittent fasting component of the plan, your last meal of the day should be no later than 6pm. This will help ease you into fasting, and avoid senseless snacking. One of the effects of Keto is it trains your body and, let's face it, your brain, to only eat when you're hungry. As times goes by, cravings cease. We often confuse cravings with hunger, when really cravings are a learned behavior and hunger is a physiological call to refuel our energy reserves.

Timing Your Fasting Period

How you decide to incorporate your intermittent fasting time is a bit flexible. Do you tend to dive in head first, or dip your toes in the water to gauge the temperature first? Knowing that about your personality will help you determine which schedule is better for you. In talking with my editor Marisa while writing this book, I learned that what was appealing to me was not to her.

I don't like feeling in a rut, and breakfast is one of my favorite meals of the day, so for that reason having an alternate schedule, allowing me to eat breakfast just about every other day, abstaining from dinner, and the reverse on opposite days (fasting through breakfast and eating dinner) is preferable. Marisa prefers consistency, something I imagine a lot of people might want as well—to go on auto-pilot, and fast at the same time every day. I can see how both fit into certain lifestyles and mindsets, that's why there are two schedules to choose from on page 51 so you can customize the 4-week Plan to fit best with your lifestyle.

Before You Get Started

Looking at the big picture is key to long-term success in any situation. This holds especially true for major diet and lifestyle changes. Intermittent Keto throws everything you thought you knew about how to eat, what to eat, and when to eat it out the window. It's not a "leap without looking" kind of decision, so it's important to familiarize yourself with what to expect, how to handle potential challenges, and how to reorganize your life in a way that enables you to achieve your goals *before* starting out.

Define Your Goals

Why did you decide to try Intermittent Keto? Is it for health reasons? Weight loss? Are you looking to just feel better and increase your energy levels? Is this meant to be a short-term detox or are you looking to make long-term lifestyle changes? How do you plan to keep track of your macronutrients? Do you plan to test for ketones to ensure you've reached a state of ketosis? Are you vegetarian or vegan?

All are important questions to consider before getting started so you can stay focused on achieving your goal. Research suggests that intermittent fasting can have profound long-term benefits. The verdict is still out on the benefits or any potential risks of implementing a Keto diet permanently. The rigidity of the plan also dictates the length of time people adhere to it.

The way you currently eat is also a big consideration when undertaking Keto, and understanding how big a change or challenge that might pose. Keto is a fat-focused diet, macronutrient-wise, but protein plays an important role. Too little protein can cause muscle loss during ketosis. Too much can kick you out of ketosis. It's a balance, and while Keto is not a high-protein diet, the default protein is often meat because plant-based protein alternatives typically are too high in carbs compared to their ratio of fiber and protein, specifically beans, including tofu which is made from soybeans.

This doesn't mean it's impossible to stay vegetarian on Keto, especially if you're an ovo-lacto vegetarian (okay with eating eggs and dairy). Non-meat protein sources that are not legumes include eggs, nuts and seeds, and cheese. The recipes in this book are geared towards an omnivorous diet. Meat plays a role in many of the recipes. If you are vegetarian, you'll need to customize your meal plan, supplementing it with recipes from outside sources. The rest of the information included in this book will be extremely helpful, and this applies to vegans, too. If you want to give Intermittent Keto a try with a vegan diet, it is not impossible but it will require even more careful planning to make sure you don't kick yourself out of ketosis by choosing protein sources too high in carbs. Many of the recipes in this book will need adjusting for your dietary needs, as well.

Testing for ketosis can be done three ways: urine test strips, blood ketone test (with a meter similar to the kind used to test blood glucose levels), and a breath test (different from Keto breath which is discussed separately). Urine tests are considered the least effective, although they are the least expensive, with blood meters considered the most accurate, and as you might've guessed, most costly.

The real question is do you need to test for ketones? If your goal is to lose weight, and the pounds are dropping, plus you feel good (well rested and energetic) after the initial few weeks, testing for ketosis might be a moot point. The more important consideration when it comes to counting numbers is monitoring what you're eating.

Why are you trying Intermittent Keto and what are your goals?

_____

_____

_____

_____

_____

_____

_____

_____

_____

_____

Take a look at this whenever you are in need of motivation.

Macronutrients vs. Calories: Which Do You Count?

Tracking your macronutrients is different from counting just calories. On Keto the emphasis is on monitoring the amount of fat, protein, and carbohydrates you consume—all macronutrients have a specific calorie count:

1 gram of fat = 9 calories
1 gram protein = 4 calories
1 gram carbohydrate = 4 calories

Counting macronutrients sounds harder than it is. Really, it's just closer scrutiny of each calorie consumed. It's still necessary to get a baseline metabolic rate, also referred to as BMR, to determine how many calories you should eat for weight maintenance and weight loss (another reason why defining your goals is important).

All of these macronutrients play a vital role in both your overall health, achieving and staying in ketosis, but the one that gets the most scrutiny on Keto is carbohydrate because it results in glucose after metabolism, which is the energy source you're trying to steer your body away from using. Some research shows the actual amount of total carbs one can consume daily on Keto is 50 grams or less, which depending on the fiber content results in 20 to 35 grams net carbs per day. The lower you can get the net carbs down, the faster your body will go into ketosis, and it'll be easier to stay in it.

Keeping in mind that we're aiming for 20 grams of net carbs a day, the fat and protein grams are variables depending on how many calories you need to consume based on your BMR. The recommended daily average for women varies between 1,600 and 2,000 calories for weight maintenance depending on level of activity (ranging from active to sedentary). Adhering to a daily plan of consuming 160 grams fat + 70 grams protein + 20 grams carbohydrates, equals 1,800 calories, and the ideal amount according to the USDA for weight maintenance for moderately active women (walking 1.5 to 3 miles a day). Based on a sedentary lifestyle, defined as only exercising as a result of normal everyday activities like cleaning and walking short distances during the course of your day, you'd want to aim for 130 grams fat + 60 grams protein + 20 grams carbohydrates to jumpstart weight loss (1,500 calories). There are plenty of online calculators to figure out your BMR, overall calorie goal, and the right ratio of fat and protein, while keeping net carbs to 20 grams per day.

Speaking of calculators and tracking numbers, you might find it helpful to establish a tracking method for your macronutrients from the recipes in this book to help customize your own unique menu. It can be as easy as writing it down in a notebook, and doing the math, but that might be more time-consuming. There's no shortage of apps for your phone to also make easy work of tracking macronutrients.

The Physical Side Effects of Keto

Unlike diet plans that simply limit the foods you eat for weight loss, keto goes deeper. Ketosis is about changing the way you eat to change the way your body converts what you eat into energy. The process of ketosis flips the equation from burning glucose (remember, carbs) to instead burning fat for fuel. This comes with possible side effects as your body adjusts to a new way of functioning. This is also why the 4-week Plan on page 53 phases in intermittent fasting during week two, and not from the get-go. It's important to give yourself time, both physically and mentally, to properly transition. Two physical changes you may experience when transitioning to a Keto diet are Keto flu and Keto breath.

Keto Flu

Keto flu, sometimes called carb flu, can last anywhere from a few days to a few weeks. Metabolic changes happening within, as your body weans itself from burning glucose for energy, may result in heightened feelings of lethargy, irritability, muscle soreness, light-headedness or brain fog, change in bowel movements, nausea, stomachaches, and trouble focusing and concentrating. I know, it sounds terrible, and probably vaguely familiar. Yes, these are all common symptoms of the flu, hence the name Keto flu.

The good news is this is a temporary phase as your body adjusts, and it doesn't affect everyone. Factors causing these symptoms include an imbalance of electrolytes (sodium, potassium, magnesium, and calcium) and sugar withdrawal from the significantly decreased carbohydrate consumption. Expecting these possible symptoms means you can be prepared to alleviate them, and decrease the length of Keto flu, should it occur at all.

Sodium levels are directly impacted by the amount of highly processed foods you consume. To clarify, everything we eat is technically a processed food, the term in itself means "a series of steps performed to achieve a particular end." Even cooking at home, from scratch, requires the act of processing food. Relating to our current culture, though, where ready-to-eat foods are at every turn in the supermarket, these highly processed foods tend to contain exorbitant levels of hidden salt (sodium is a preservative as well as a flavor enhancer).

Adhering to a Keto diet is most successful when you're doing the actual cooking, where you can control the amount of carbs and hidden sugars in a dish. Home cooking tends to be less processed, which might also result in lower sodium. Increasing the amount of salt in your food, and drinking a homemade stock like the Bone Broth on page 127 is an easy, natural way to boost your sodium levels.

Below are other foods to focus on during your Keto phase-in. They're naturally rich in magnesium, potassium, and calcium to help keep electrolytes in balance.

Magnesium (helps with muscle soreness and leg cramps)
    Avocados
    broccoli
    fish
    kale
    almonds
    pumpkin seeds
    spinach

Potassium (helps with muscle soreness, hydration)
    Asparagus
    avocados
    Brussels sprouts
    salmon
    tomatoes
    leafy greens

*Calcium (especially important if you were a big
milk drinker pre-keto!)*
   Almonds
   bok choy
   broccoli
   cheese
   collard greens
   spinach
   sardines
   sesame and chia seeds

Another way to possibly ward off the chances of
experiencing Keto flu is to begin slowly decreasing
your carb intake a few weeks before starting the
4-week Plan. It can be as simple as swapping your
morning muffin for hard-boiled or scrambled eggs,
skipping the bun and wrapping your burger in lettuce
(often referred to as protein-style when ordering), or
swapping out spaghetti for courgetti. This way when
you dive into the plan on page 51 it'll feel more
like a natural progression to eating less carbs than
a sharp right turn.

Keto Breath

Let's cut to the chase here. Bad breath stinks, literally, but it's something you should brace yourself for
when switching to Keto. There's two thoughts as to
why this occurs.

As your body enters ketosis, and begins releasing ketones (a by-product of burning fat for fuel), one of the ketones released is acetone (yes, the same solvent found in nail polish remover and paint thinners). Acetone is excreted through urine and from your breath in the body's attempt to finish the metabolic process of breaking down those fatty acids. This can also result in unpleasant-smelling breath as the acetone is released.

Protein can also be a factor contributing to Keto breath. Remember, the macronutrient goal is high fat, moderate protein, and low carb. People often think high fat is interchangeable with high protein. On the contrary, that is far from true. The body digests fat and protein differently. Our bodies produce ammonia when breaking down protein, and usually release it during urine output. Eating more protein than you need results in the undigested amount lingering in your gut where it ferments, producing ammonia, which is then released through your breath.

The upside is Keto breath is a good indicator your body is in ketosis. How long the smell lasts varies according to how well your body adapts to ketosis. Many sources indicate it lasts anywhere from one week to less than a month. A deeper dig through Keto message boards and chat groups shows it can persist for months, while some people report never experiencing it. Some solutions to possibly avoid or lessen Keto breath are to always be armed with sugar-free gum, reduce your protein intake, make sure you stick to a good dental routine (brushing and flossing), and following the advice mentioned earlier on about gradually reducing your carbohydrate intake before jumping full steam ahead into the 4-week Plan.

Sleep & Exercise

Every healthy lifestyle includes adequate sleep and moderate activity. The same advice should be considered when defining your goals, and figuring out how both fit into your daily routine. Once you incorporate intermittent fasting into your plan, those sleeping hours become even more necessary since they're part of your fasting time. Keep mindless late-night snacking urges at bay by tucking in at a reasonable hour.

Weight training is a big focus among Keto enthusiasts, and it's certainly important when you're in maintenance mode. When it comes to weight loss, cardio workouts provide the biggest fat-burning benefit. Be sure to consult your doctor before making any major changes if you have underlying health concerns.

Talk With Your Friends & Family

Mention the word diet, and you'll find most people have strong opinions that increase in intensity depending on which plan you choose to follow. Everyone is entitled to their opinions, and sharing similar experiences is sometimes helpful when you're looking for inspiration or motivation. What's not beneficial is people who say "you look fine the way you are" or "I could never give up carbs", or worse "you're going to starve yourself!"

Every ship needs a captain to steer it, so consider yourself the captain of your body. Friends and family should be there to support you on this journey, so empower them with the information to do so. Let them know why you're making the switch if you're comfortable talking about it. At the very least, explain the principles behind why intermittent fasting and Keto work really well for some people. Often people are simply wary of what they don't know, and don't take the time to seek out answers. You can even give them a copy of this book if they want to look deeper into it, too. You never know if you'll inspire someone to try Intermittent Keto, too, and then you'll have a buddy to track progress with, set goals, and keep each other motivated.

Sharing your decision to go on Keto is also a good way to avoid showing up at a friend's dinner party to find they're only serving pasta. If you are going over to a friend's you could volunteer to bring a course to share that's also Keto-friendly for you to enjoy. This way it alleviates any stress they might have about cooking for you, plus it highlights some of the amazing foods you can eat on Keto!

There will be those who think they know better, or insist it's okay to cheat here and there. Maybe that works for other diets, but you can easily knock yourself out of ketosis by consuming too many carbohydrates. Be a good advocate for yourself, and don't be afraid to say "no thank you". Anyone who truly cares about you will respect the hard work you're putting in to develop a healthier lifestyle for yourself without trying to tempt you.

Obviously, you also want to keep your intermittent fasting schedule in mind when you're making plans. Late night dinners don't really jive, but you can meet for drinks, and keep your order to a plain seltzer with a lime wedge, or better yet, meet for coffee post dinner. The 4-week Plan was designed to give you a break from intermittent fasting on Sunday mornings, since it's a popular time to gather with friends, and brunch is very easy to stick to on the Keto diet.

Staying In Ketosis & What Happens If You Fall Out Of It

Once you enter ketosis, how long you decide to stick with it is up to you after you finish the 4-week Plan. Was your goal simply to drop a dress size? A month may be all you need. Were you trying to wean yourself off sugar, or reduce your overall carb intake? Perhaps a little longer might be good to help establish long-term eating patterns even after you decide to increase your total carb count beyond the 20 grams per day allotted in the 4-week Plan. Technically anything less than 50 grams of carbohydrates (overall, not net carbs) helps kick your body into fat burning mode, so even a minor increase in carbs can offer a mild ketosis benefit, though you might regain back a few of the pounds you initially lost.

Be prepared for learning curves, and possible pitfalls. It's possible to kick your body out of ketosis if you eat too much protein, too many carbs, or don't get enough exercise. A simple mistake, or just giving into a craving, such as eating a sweet potato, can put you back into glucose-burning mode. If Keto sounds strict, that's because it is. Getting into ketosis and maintaining it is a commitment, which is why we talked about defining your goals early on. While it might seem disastrous or frustrating after all the hard work you put in, don't beat yourself up. Focus on your future goals, and getting yourself back into ketosis. Don't extend the cheat, thinking "oh, well, the damage is done." Instead, fasting after a cheat day is one way to get yourself back on track, keeping in mind you'll have to burn through that glucose again first.

Journaling, in general, is a great way to track more than just calories. Start recording how you're feeling physically, and your mental outlook—a simple number-rating system helps you understand if you're making progress, maintaining status quo, or slipping with your goals. Detailed notes might help pinpoint more direct reasons related to your cheat day to help plan better in the future. In fact, it might be the case that you'll want to plan for the occasional cheat day, instead of beating yourself up for them after. If you know your best friend's wedding is coming up, and you want to partake 100% in the festivities, including all the food and drink served, plan for that. While you can't just flip a switch to get back into ketosis, you'll know what to expect, and hopefully get back on track quicker than the first time. It's also worth mentioning that you shouldn't rely on too many cheat days. Again, this ties back to defining your goals.

Know What Foods To Enjoy & What Foods To Avoid

It's so easy to think about what you can't eat on Keto, but it's much more fun to focus on all things you *can* enjoy. Here's a chart you can reference when you're in need of some inspiration.

Keto Cheat Sheet

EAT	AVOID
Courgetti, spaghetti squash & shirataki noodles	Pasta
Use almond flour, unsweetened coconut flakes & pork cracklings	Breadcrumbs
Cauliflower rice, Shirataki rice	Rice, couscous
Double cream & cheeses (mozzarella, cheddar)	Milk
Low-carb tortillas & keto bread (see page 129)	Bread, wraps, tortillas
Pureed Cauliflower	Mashed potatoes
Courgette Fries (see page 142)	French Fries & Sweet Potato Fries
Berries, use lemons & limes for flavor	Sweet citrus (oranges, grapefruit, clementines), tropical fruits (bananas, mango, pineapple), all dried fruits
Meat, poultry, seafood, eggs	Beans, tofu
Stevia, monkfruit	Sweeteners (honey, maple syrup, sugar)
Olive oil, coconut oil, avocado oil, butter, ghee, sesame oil (in small quantities)	Sunflower, grapeseed, canola, peanut, safflower oils, margarine, vegetable shortening
Parmesan Crisps (see page 137)	Potato crisps & sweet/salty snacks
Water (key for staying hydrated), coffee, tea	Sugary drinks, (soda, juices), alcohol

The Keto Kitchen

Leading up to starting Intermittent Keto, it's important to make sure your pantry aligns with your new eating goals. Those new goals might be at odds with the rest of the members of your household, be they family or roommates. If so, clearing out all the carb-laden foods, sugary snacks, and processed foods might not be a possibility. It'll be an exercise in self-control, especially the first week or two when cravings might be tricky to manage. Don't fret. You can still claim an area of the kitchen and set up a Keto-friendly zone to make sticking to the plan easier. And by all means, if you live on your own, or your partner/family is doing this with you, go full throttle, and use an "out with the old, in with the new" approach. Instead of discarding unwanted items, donate them to a local food bank (check expiration dates first), or to your neighbors.

Once you've got a clean slate, it's time to start filling the pantry with all the foods you can enjoy. Here are staple ingredients you'll want to add to your first shopping list.

Fermented foods (make sure veggies are lacto-fermented):
   pickles
   kimchi
   sauerkraut
   plain full-fat yogurt

Oils:
    avocado oil
    extra virgin olive oil
    cold-pressed or virgin coconut oil
    ghee
    MCT oil

Nuts & Seeds (and flours made from them):
    almonds
    walnuts
    macadamia nuts
    Brazil nuts
    pecans
    chia seeds
    pumpkin seeds
    sunflower seeds
    sesame seeds
    almond flour or meal
    coconut flour

Canned goods & other shelf-stable items
(make sure all nut milks are unsweetened):
    coconut cream
    coconut milk
    almond milk
    olives
    dark chocolate (Lily's dark chocolate chips are
        sweetened with stevia)
    cocoa powder

tea & coffee (plain, unflavored)
pork rinds
baking powder (see note below)

Spices & Sweeteners:
red pepper flakes
basil
oregano
bay leaves
smoked paprika
sea salt
black pepper
cumin
curry powder
everything bagel seasoning
wholegrain mustard
stevia
monk fruit sweetener (read label to make sure it's
    not a blend mixed with sugar)

Perishables:
bacon and sausage (be sure to buy sugar-free
    varieties)
eggs
coconut wraps
low-carb tortillas
sugar-free mayonnaise
double cream
butter
cheese

A Word About Baking Powder & Other Ingredients

One look at the ingredients, and you'll notice there's cornstarch in commercial baking powder. It's actually in most homemade recipes, too. Baking powder is traditionally made with a combination of baking soda, cream of tartar, and cornstarch. Some Keto folks will tell you cornstarch is absolutely forbidden since it's a grain, and you're not supposed to eat any grains on Keto. It's important to remember why you're not supposed to eat grains, though, before settling on a conclusion about baking powder. The underlying reason is because grains are carb-heavy, and Keto is a low-carb diet. The reality is, the amount of cornstarch in baking powder compared to how much you actually use in a recipe is so negligible, it barely registers. If you're grain free for health reasons, then that's a good reason to make your own baking powder, or seek out a brand without any (I've yet to find one that exists, but that may change by the printing of this book). All of the recipes in this book were tested using store-bought baking powder. Results using a homemade version without cornstarch aren't guaranteed.

Most bacon has sugar added during the curing process, even from small, artisanal farmers. While the actual amount of sugar in the end product is minimal, you might want to look for a brand that has no sugar added if you're having trouble balancing your carb count.

Not all ketchups are created equal. In fact, many are loaded with sugar. Be sure to buy an unsweetened brand like Primal Kitchen for dipping and to make the BBQ sauce on page 82.

Many Keto enthusiasts swear by MCT oil. It's not coconut oil, but rather a by-product of coconut. MCT stands for medium chain triglycerides. Among the health benefits it supposedly offers are keeping you satiated (feeling full), providing a quick boost of energy, and supporting a healthy immune system. The full feeling it offers may be why some people believe it aids in weight loss, preventing you from overeating or snacking.

Weekly Grocery Shopping

When it comes to produce, all herbs get a green light—great news since they're easy flavor boosters to any meal. The general rule of thumb for vegetables is stick to ones that grow above ground. That means steer clear of root vegetables and tubers (think carrots, parsnips, beets, onions, regular and sweet potatoes) as they're starchier vegetables, higher in carbohydrates. Some above-ground vegetables are high-carb, too, such as winter squash, pumpkin, corn, and peas.

You can still eat the rainbow, so don't worry— dark leafy greens (kale, spinach), broccoli, cauliflower, courgettes (courgetti!), radishes, cucumbers, garlic, asparagus, mushrooms, and eggplant all make the list for Keto meals.

Fruit lovers might find Keto challenging since most are too high in natural sugars, and therefore off limits, especially dried fruits which have higher concentrations of sugar. Your choices are basically berries, since they're mostly fiber, lemon and limes. All other citrus fruit is too high in natural sugars, but guess what? If you love orange essence in some dishes, you can use orange zest to add flavor without the carbs!

At this point, you might feel weighed down by all the things you can't eat. That's a normal feeling, and while it's a reality if you're committed to Keto, I always prefer to focus on the foods I can eat, so snap a photo of that Keto Cheat Sheet on page 37, and you'll always have a quick reference point when in doubt.

Essential Kitchen Tools

Veteran cooks likely have a well-stocked kitchen. If you're just starting out, you'll quickly realize cooking your own food increases your success with sticking to a Keto diet. Here's a list of kitchen tools and equipment you'll find helpful in preparing meals. I tend to stay away from gadgets that only serve one purpose, but exceptions to that rule are my spiralizer and avocado slicer. Homemade courgetti is a breeze to make with my hand-held spiralizer. You can pick one up for less than £10.

Avocados are a Keto fan favorite. Pitting avocados also results in more emergency room visits than you might imagine, and can result in nerve damage. This actually happened to a dear friend who's an experienced cook. She now owns an avocado slicer.

Regarding frying pans, I find non-stick to be great if you can only buy one set of pans. Even though you'll be using considerably more fat in your cooking than you currently use, nonstick frying pans are great for making eggs and pancakes (check out the Blueberry Almond Pancakes on page 63!).

8-inch frying pan
10-inch frying pan
Spiralizer
Digital kitchen scale
Bento box for packing lunches
Tongs & spatula
Avocado slicer
Mason jars (for preparing and transporting chia puddings)
Silicon candy molds (for making fat bombs)
Chef's knife & paring knife

Variety of pots (ranging from 2-quarts to 8-quarts, if space and budget permit)
Cutting boards
Blender
Food processor (optional, but especially helpful to grind your own nut flours)

When To Stop & How To Stop: How Long Should You Continue Keto and Intermittent Fasting?

We've one last thing to discuss before you dive into your 4-week Plan. It ties somewhat into your defined goals. Keto is strict on *what* you can and cannot eat. Throw in intermittent fasting, and now you restrict *when* you can eat. This is also a good time to talk about how long you should, or want, to stay on Keto. Currently, there isn't enough research to make a conclusion from a health perspective as to Keto's long term efficacy, but the truth is you're fighting your body's natural instinct to fuel itself on glucose. Even though we evolved under the premise of fat for fuel, times changed, and along with it so did our bodies for better or worse.

Even though the research is lacking to provide any concrete theories, besides those related to underlying medical issues, many people lean towards using Keto a few times a year for a prolonged period of time, anywhere from a few weeks, to a couple of months, taking a break in between, but still being mindful of overall carb consumption.

Intermittent fasting is a different story. I know someone who's been intermittent fasting for a few years now. She does it differently than the plan outlined here, and is not on Keto, so her experience is different, but intermittent fasting has been very successful and manageable for her to maintain. She's also one of the biggest foodies and cooks I know. Intermittent fasting hasn't cramped her style one bit. Quite the opposite. She actually looks forward to her fast days as they leave her feeling refreshed and focused. Should you decide to step away from the Keto diet, and stay with intermittent fasting, I suggest doing some research to figure out the best method and schedule for yourself.

When you feel you've reached the end of your Keto journey, or just want to press pause for a duration beyond a cheat, you must do it in a meaningful and methodical way. Remember it took time for your body to adjust to ketosis. Same goes for reverting back to a diet that has more carbohydrates which will flip the switch back to burning glucose for energy. This applies even if your plan is to stay on a lower-carb diet than you ate before starting Keto.

Things to keep in mind when deciding to switch off Keto are:

- Take it slow, introducing more carbs a little at a time.
- Expect some weight gain. The amount depends on how long you've been on Keto. The early weeks of weight loss on keto tend to be water weight. If you've been on Keto for a while, the weight gain should be less provided you're not overindulging in carbs and sugar.
- Familiarize yourself with healthy portion sizes again, adjusting the quantity of fats and proteins accordingly.

Part II

Meal Plans and Recipes

Ready, Set, Go: 4-week Plan & Recipes

Weekend Before

Saturday
Clean out the pantry. Make shopping lists.

Sunday
Go grocery shopping—stick to the perimeter of the supermarket, all the super processed items tend to be clustered in the middle aisles. Prep food for the week ahead.

4-week Plan

How you decide to work in your fasting time depends on whether you would prefer to follow the same structure each day or whether you like to mix things up a bit. Whichever approach you opt for, remember that IF is only introduced in week two. This first plan has you fasting at the same time each day and allows for one day a week without fasting expecting you might want to enjoy a Sunday brunch with friends (keto foods only). If you want, you can omit Sunday brunch to stick with your IF routine. Just be sure to include a mid-afternoon snack to make sure you consume your necessary macronutrients. The second plan has you fasting on alternate days so you'll abstain from breakfast and eat dinner every other day and the reverse on opposite days. In the Resources section at the back of the book, you'll find blank meal planners for the full 4 weeks so you can plot out your recipes for the weeks ahead.

4-week Meals Noon to 6pm Only

Week 1	Monday	Tuesday	Wednesday	Thursday	Friday	Saturday	Sunday
Morning	KETO	KETO	KETO	KETO	KETO	FAST	FAST
Noon	KETO	KETO	KETO	KETO	KETO	KETO	KETO
Before 6pm	KETO	KETO	KETO	KETO	KETO	KETO	KETO
Week 2							
Morning	FAST	FAST	FAST	FAST	FAST	FAST	KETO
Noon	KETO	KETO	KETO	KETO	KETO	KETO	KETO
Midday Snack	KETO	KETO	KETO	KETO	KETO	KETO	none
Before 6pm	KETO	KETO	KETO	KETO	KETO	KETO	KETO
Week 3							
Morning	FAST	FAST	FAST	FAST	FAST	FAST	KETO
Noon	KETO	KETO	KETO	KETO	KETO	KETO	KETO
Midday Snack	KETO	KETO	KETO	KETO	KETO	KETO	none
Before 6pm	KETO	KETO	KETO	KETO	KETO	KETO	KETO
Week 4							
Morning	FAST	FAST	FAST	FAST	FAST	FAST	KETO
Noon	KETO	KETO	KETO	KETO	KETO	KETO	KETO
Midday Snack	KETO	KETO	KETO	KETO	KETO	KETO	none
Before 6pm	KETO	KETO	KETO	KETO	KETO	KETO	KETO

4-week Plan – Alternate Intermittent Fasting

Week 1	Monday	Tuesday	Wednesday	Thursday	Friday	Saturday	Sunday
Morning	KETO	KETO	KETO	KETO	KETO	FAST	KETO
Noon	KETO	KETO	KETO	KETO	KETO	KETO	KETO
Before 6pm	KETO	KETO	KETO	KETO	KETO	KETO	FAST
Week 2							
Morning	KETO	KETO	FAST	KETO	FAST	KETO	KETO
Noon	KETO	KETO	KETO	KETO	KETO	KETO	KETO
Before 6pm	FAST	FAST	KETO	FAST	KETO	KETO	FAST
Week 3							
Morning	FAST	KETO	FAST	KETO	FAST	KETO	KETO
Noon	KETO	KETO	KETO	KETO	KETO	KETO	KETO
Before 6pm	KETO	FAST	KETO	FAST	KETO	KETO	FAST
Week 4							
Morning	FAST	KETO	FAST	KETO	FAST	KETO	KETO
Noon	KETO	KETO	KETO	KETO	KETO	KETO	KETO
Before 6pm	KETO	FAST	KETO	FAST	KETO	KETO	FAST

Cookbooks are generally broken into traditional categories of breakfast, lunch, dinner, treats and beverages. You'll find the recipe table of contents and menu plans on pages 7 to 9 set up that way for familiarity. Since keto is all about focusing on your macronutrients, what really matters is eating the right ratios of fat, protein, and carbs. Keeping that in mind, feel free to swap out breakfast for lunch, lunch for dinner, or even dinner for breakfast. Just track your macros to make sure you don't overeat any of them.

BREAKFAST

Pecan & Coconut N'oatmeal

Bacon, Egg & Cheese Breakfast "Muffins"

Herb & Cheddar Baked Avocado Eggs

Blueberry Almond Pancakes

Toad in the Hole

Berry Breakfast Shake

Cheddar, Spinach & Mushroom Omelette

Pecan & Coconut N'Oatmeal

Serves 1

This is a hearty breakfast porridge for cold mornings when you're craving a steaming bowl of oatmeal, but without the carb overload.

Calories	312
Fat	5
Protein	13.4
Carbs	7
Fiber	5
Net carbs	2

½ cup coconut or almond milk
2 teaspoons chia seeds
2 tablespoons almond flour
1 tablespoon ground flaxseed
2 tablespoons hemp seeds
¼ teaspoon ground cinnamon
¼ teaspoon pure vanilla extract
1 tablespoon pecans, toasted & chopped
1 tablespoon coconut flakes

In a small pot, combine the milk, chia seeds, almond flour, ground flaxseed, hemp seeds, cinnamon, and vanilla.

Cook over low heat, stirring constantly until thickened, about 5 minutes. Spoon into a bowl, top with the pecans and coconut flakes, and enjoy immediately.

Bacon, Egg & Cheese Breakfast "Muffins"

Makes 6

These breakfast muffins are basically a bacon, egg and cheese sandwich without the bread. They're incredibly portable for busy mornings, so make a batch on the weekends, and you'll have a quick grab 'n' go breakfast during the week (heat them in the microwave for 30 to 60 seconds). The recipe is a blank canvas of sorts. Feel free to add any leftover cooked veggies in the fridge, fresh herbs, or swap in ham for the bacon.

Calories	303
Fat	26
Protein	15
Carbs	1.5
Fiber	0
Net carbs	1.5

6 slices bacon
8 eggs
¼ cup double cream
Fine sea salt and freshly ground black pepper, to taste
3 ounces Cheddar cheese, shredded

Preheat the oven to 375°F (190°C). Generously grease the

bottoms and sides of a 6-cup muffin tin (softened butter works best for this).

Add the bacon to a cold 10-inch frying pan, and place over medium-high heat. Cook until crisp all over, turning once. Transfer to a paper-towel lined plate. Crumble the bacon into pieces.

In a deep bowl, whisk together the eggs, cream, salt, and pepper.

Sprinkle an even amount of cheese and bacon into each cup of the prepared tin. Pour an even amount of egg mixture over the filling.

Bake 20 to 25 minutes, until the eggs puff up, and are lightly golden.

Herb & Cheddar Baked Avocado Eggs

Serves 2

A delicious, hearty savoury dish, perfect for lunch or supper. The combination of cheese and avocado make it very satisfying and will lessen your desire to cheat!

Calories	257
Fat	22
Protein	13
Carbs	1.3
Fiber	0
Net carbs	1.3

2 eggs
2 ounces Cheddar cheese, shredded
2 teaspoons double cream
1 teaspoon fresh chopped chives
Sea salt and freshly ground black pepper, to taste
1 avocado, cut in half and pitted (see Note)

Preheat the oven to 425°F (220°C).

Combine the eggs, cheese, cream, half the chives, salt, and pepper in a medium bowl. Beat with a fork until well mixed.

Arrange the avocado halves in a small rimmed baking

dish, cut side up (they should be snug so they don't roll around). Pour the egg filling into the center of each avocado.

Bake 12 minutes, until the filling is lightly golden on top. Serve hot topped with the remaining chives.

Note: Avocado pits vary, so depending on the size, you might need to scoop a little bit extra avocado from the center with a spoon to accommodate the egg filling.

Blueberry Almond Pancakes

Makes 10 to 12 (serving size two pancakaes)

Aside from the lack of grains, these pancakes are different in another way—you cover the pan with a lid while they're cooking to ensure they cook through in the center.

Calories	114
Fat	10
Protein	3.9
Carbs	3.9
Fiber	1.4
Net carbs	2.5

4 tablespoons butter, plus extra to cook the pancakes
2 large eggs
¼ cup almond milk
¼ teaspoon pure vanilla extract
¾ cup almond flour
1 tablespoon ground flaxseed
1 teaspoon baking powder
1 packet stevia powder
¼ teaspoon sea salt
¼ teaspoon allspice (optional)
¾ cup blueberries, frozen or fresh

In a small bowl, whisk the 4 tablespoons of butter, eggs, almond milk, and vanilla. Whisk in the flour, ground flax-seed baking powder, stevia, salt, and allspice until well blended. Fold in the blueberries.

Heat a nonstick frying pan over medium heat. It's ready to use when a few drops of water dance across the surface. Melt a pat of butter in the pan. Drop scant ¼ cupfuls of batter into the frying pan, spreading out into thin circles (they'll puff up). Cover the pan with a lid, and cook for 1 to 2 minutes until air bubbles appear on top and the batter has firmed up slightly. Flip, and fry until cooked through and golden underneath, about 2 minutes more. Serve hot.

Note: Leftover pancakes may be layered between parchment paper, wrapped in clingfilm and stored in the freezer for up 1 month. Heat them straight from the freezer in a 350°F (180°C) oven for 8 to 10 minutes.

Toad in the Hole

Serves 2

A Keto version of a traditional family favourite. Use beet sausages if you prefer.

Calories	376
Fat	28
Protein	16.3
Carbs	16.2
Fiber	2.4
Net carbs	13.8

4 pork sausages (spicy or sweet)
⅓ cup blanched fine almond flour
3 tablespoons arrowroot
6 tablespoons almond milk
¼ cup double cream
1 egg
¼ teaspoon sea salt

Place an 8-inch cast iron frying pan on the center rack of the oven. Preheat oven to 400°F (200°C).

Place the sausages in the pan. Cook, turning once, until nicely browned, 12 to 15 minutes.

Meanwhile, combine the almond flour, arrowroot,

almond milk, cream, egg, and salt in a medium bowl. Whisk until mixed well.

Once the sausages are browned, remove the pan and pour the batter into it. Return the pan to the oven, and cook until puffed up and golden, 20 to 25 minutes. Serve immediately.

Berry Breakfast Shake

Serves 1

This is the perfect quick, easy but delicious start to the day. Especially for breakfast on the run!

Calories	900
Fat	80
Protein	10
Carbs	18
Fiber	5
Net carbs	13

¼ cup frozen mixed berries
½ cup double cream
½ cup coconut or almond milk
1 tablespoon almond butter
½ teaspoon freshly squeezed lemon juice
1 tablespoon MCT oil (optional)

Place all the ingredients in a blender bowl. Blend until smooth. Serve immediately.

Cheddar, Spinach & Mushroom Omelette

Serves 2

Sure, this recipe is included the breakfast category, but omelettes are also a great go-to meal for lunch and dinner, so keep that in mind when planning your menu for the week.

Calories	500
Fat	38
Protein	34
Carbs	5
Fiber	1
Net carbs	4

2 teaspoons extra virgin olive oil
3 ounces white button mushrooms, sliced
2 packed cups baby spinach
Sea salt, to taste
Handful of fresh parsley, chopped
6 large eggs, lightly beaten
4 ounces Cheddar cheese, shredded

In an 8-inch nonstick frying pan, heat 1 teaspoon of oil over a medium-high heat until shimmering. Add the mushrooms. Cook, shaking the pan a few times, until the mushrooms are golden, 3 to 4 minutes. Stir in the spinach, and season with salt. Cook until just wilted, 1 to 2 minutes. Transfer the vegetables to a bowl. Stir in the parsley; set aside. Heat the remaining teaspoon of oil in the same pan. Season the eggs with salt, and pour into the pan. Cook, without disturbing the eggs, until the edges are set. Using a rubber spatula, lift underneath the edges of the egg while tilting the pan so any uncooked egg can slide underneath and cook. Cover one half of the eggs with the vegetable mixture. Sprinkle the cheese on top. Fold the plain egg over the half with the vegetables, to create a half moon. Cook for 1 minute more. Serve immediately.

LUNCH

Bacon, Avocado & Turkey Lettuce Wraps

Spicy Sesame Courgetti

Italian Stuffed Peppers

Warm Spinach & Roast Chicken Salad
with Bacon Vinaigrette

Chicken Caesar Salad with Parmesan Crisps

Buffalo Chicken Wings with Ranch Dipping Sauce

Bacon & Shrimp Lollipops

Shrimp & Avocado Cobb Salad

Pork Fried Cauliflower Couscous

Bacon, Avocado & Turkey Lettuce Wraps

Serves 2

Cooking up a batch of bacon, and keeping it in the fridge makes for fast weekday lunches. A quick reheat in a frying pan is enough to crisp it up. Feel free to swap in leftover roast chicken in place of turkey.

Calories	510
Fat	44
Protein	17
Carbs	14.6
Fiber	7.3
Net carbs	7.3

2 large lettuce leaves
1 tablespoon mayonnaise
4 slices cooked bacon
1 avocado, pitted and sliced
4 slices turkey

Lay each lettuce leaf on a board. Brush with the mayonnaise. On one half of each, layer two pieces of bacon, half the avocado slices, and two slices of turkey. Roll up starting with the end that's filled. Enjoy.

Spicy Sesame Courgetti

Serves 2

Cold sesame noodles used to be a favorite lunch of mine. Here, I'm swapping in Courgette noodles (Courgetti page 141). The sauce traditionally has a sweetener to balance out the heaviness of the almond butter. I've opted to leave it out here, but if you'd prefer, you can add ½ a packet of stevia to the dressing as you whisk it together in the bowl.

Calories	507
Fat	47.6
Protein	12.9
Carbs	14
Fiber	6.8
Net carbs	7.2

1 lime, cut in half
¼ cup smooth almond butter
1 tablespoon soy sauce
1 tablespoon sesame oil
½ teaspoon red pepper chilli flakes
Sea salt, to taste
½ cup shredded red cabbage
Handful fresh coriander, leaves and stems chopped
2 spring onions, chopped
⅓ cup sliced almonds
Courgetti (page 141)

Juice half the lime into a deep bowl. Cut the remaining lime in half; set aside.

Add the almond butter, soy sauce, sesame oil, and chilli flakes to the bowl. Season with salt. Whisk until well blended.

Add the cabbage, coriander, spring onions, almonds, and Courgetti to the bowl. Toss to coat. Serve immediately, or chill until serving.

Italian Stuffed Peppers

Serves 2

We all know the benefits of the Mediterranean diet. This Italian-inspired Keto dish will make you feel as if you are on holiday in Tuscany.

Calories	574
Fat	40.2
Protein	36.8
Carbs	17.9
Fiber	4.2
Net carbs	13.7

1 tablespoon extra virgin olive oil
8 ounces ground beef
1 garlic clove, chopped
1 cup Slow-Simmered Tomato Sauce (page 132)
½ teaspoon dried basil
½ teaspoon dried oregano
Sea salt and freshly ground black pepper
1 cup Cauliflower Couscous (page 139)
4 ounces mozzarella, shredded
2 red bell peppers

In a medium frying pan, add the oil and heat until shimmering. Add the beef, and use a fork to break up any chunks (you want little bits of meat). Season with salt and pepper. Cook until well browned. Use a slotted spoon to transfer to a bowl; set aside.

Add the garlic to the pan. Sauté until fragrant, about 1 minute.

Stir in the tomato sauce, basil and oregano, then add the meat back to the pan. Season with salt and pepper. Reduce the heat to low, and simmer for 5 minutes.

Preheat the oven to 375°F (190°C).

Remove the meat filling from the heat, and let cool slightly while the oven preheats.

Stir in the Cauliflower Couscous and half the mozzarella into the filling.

Slice the tops off the bell peppers, and scoop out the seeds. Evenly spoon the meat filling into the peppers. Arrange the peppers in an 8-inch loaf tin. Sprinkle the remaining mozzarella on top.

Bake for 35 to 40 minutes, until the peppers are soft and the cheese is lightly golden. Serve hot.

Warm Spinach & Roast Chicken Salad with Bacon Vinaigrette

Serves 2

Most people add cold bacon to a hot pan, and then duck for cover from the splatter. The easiest way to avoid this is to add cold bacon to a *cold* pan (genius, right?). The drippings form the base for a flavorful dressing for what might otherwise seem a very a simple salad. Leftover chicken from making the Bone Broth on page 127 or the Smoky Butter Roast Chicken on page 101 both work well here.

Calories	489
Fat	32
Protein	43.8
Carbs	2.9
Fiber	1.3
Net carbs	1.6

4 slices bacon
1 garlic clove, smashed
2 teaspoons Dijon mustard
2 tablespoons red wine vinegar
Sea salt and freshly ground black pepper
2 cups cubed or shredded cooked chicken
4 packed cups baby spinach

Add the bacon to a cold 8-inch frying pan, and place over a medium-high heat. Cook until crisp all over, turning once. Transfer to a paper towel-lined plate.

In the same pan, add the garlic. Saute until fragrant, about 1 minute. Discard the garlic. Off the heat, whisk in the mustard and vinegar. Season with salt and pepper. Return the pan to a low flame. Stir in the chicken, and cook until warmed, 1 to 2 minutes. Remove the pan from the heat, stir in the spinach, then immediately divide the salad between two shallow bowls. Enjoy straight away.

Chicken Caesar Salad with Parmesan Crisps

Serves 2

This salad is a favorite for a few reasons. First it uses up leftover roast chicken from the recipe on page 101. If you're craving it, but don't have leftover roast chicken you can use store-bought rotisserie (stick to the herb or plain roasted ones since they likely won't have any added sugar). This is an easy lunch to pack for busy weekdays.

Calories	321
Fat	29
Protein	12.4
Carbs	2.8
Fiber	1
Net carbs	1.8

¼ cup mayonnaise
1 garlic clove
1 teaspoon freshly squeezed lemon juice
¼ teaspoon soy sauce
½ teaspoon anchovy paste
1 tablespoon grated Parmesan cheese
¼ teaspoon Dijon mustard
1 bunch romaine hearts, chopped
2 cups leftover Smoky Butter Roast Chicken
6 Parmesan Crisps (page 137)

To make the dressing, add the mayonnaise, garlic, lemon juice, soy sauce, anchovy paste, Parmesan, and mustard in a blender. Blend until the dressing is smooth and creamy. In a deep bowl, combine the lettuce and chicken. Add half of the dressing, and toss until well coated. Garnish with Parmesan Crisps. Serve immediately with the rest of the dressing on the side.

Buffalo Chicken Wings
with Ranch Dipping Sauce

Serves 2

This tasty chicken dish is incredibly quick and easy to prepare.

Calories	310
Fat	26.3
Protein	16.3
Carbs	2.4
Fiber	0.1
Net carbs	2.3

Olive oil, for greasing
1 teaspoon baking powder
½ teaspoon garlic powder
½ teaspoon black pepper, plus more as needed
¼ teaspoon sea salt, plus more as needed
8 chicken wings
2 tablespoons melted butter
¼ cup hot sauce (preferably one without added sugar)
¼ cup Homemade Ranch Dressing (page 134)

Preheat the oven to 375°F (190°C). Generously brush an 11-inch by 17-inch baking sheet with olive oil.

Combine the baking powder, garlic powder, pepper, salt, and 1 tablespoon water in a deep bowl. Add the chicken, and toss until well coated. Arrange the chicken in a single layer on the prepared sheet. Bake for 20 to 25 minutes, turning halfway through, until golden on both sides.

Meanwhile, whisk together the butter and hot sauce in a small bowl. Pour over the chicken, turning them to make sure they're well coated. Increase the oven temperature to 400°F (200°C). Bake for 10 to 15 minutes more, turning halfway through, until crispy.

Serve the chicken wings hot with the Homemade Ranch Dressing as a dipping sauce.

Bacon & Prawn Lollipops

Serves 2

This play on surf and turf is perfect party food, so keep this recipe in your back pocket whether you're hosting, or going to a friend's house.

Calories	410
Fat	34
Protein	25
Carbs	1
Fiber	0
Net carbs	1

6 slices bacon (thin-cut works best)
6 jumbo prawns, peeled and deveined
2 wooden or metal skewers (If using wooden
    skewers, soak them in water for 2 hours to avoid
    any splinters)

Preheat the grill of your oven.

Use one piece of bacon to wrap around one prawn (imagine you're looping a piece of ribbon around a ring) to cover it completely. Repeat with the remaining bacon and shrimp.

Add three pieces to each skewer, sliding the skewer

through the shrimp length ways (instead of right through the center). Place on a rimmed baking sheet.

Grill for 4 to 5 minutes, until browned. Turn and grill for 4 to 5 minutes more until cooked through. Serve hot.

Prawn & Avocado Cobb Salad

Serves 2

This makes a perfect summer lunch or light supper. Fresh and crunchy, especially when served with delicious home-made vinaigrette.

Calories	838
Fat	69.6
Protein	40
Carbs	17.9
Fiber	9.5
Net carbs	8.4

8 large prawns, peeled & deveined
1 head of Boston lettuce, chopped
1 romaine heart, chopped
10 cherry tomatoes, halved
4 hard-boiled eggs, cut in half
4 slices cooked bacon, crumbled
1 avocado, pitted and chopped
¼ cup Easy Homemade Vinaigrette (page 121)

To cook the prawns, fill a 2-quart pot with water and bring to the boil over a high heat. Add the prawns. Cover and remove the pot from heat. Set aside for 10 minutes.

Drain the prawns, and set them in a bowl of ice water to stop the cooking process; set aside.

Arrange the lettuces, tomatoes, eggs, bacon, avocado, and prawns between two shallow bowls. Drizzle the dressing on top. Serve immediately.

Note: My method for making foolproof hard-boiled eggs is to place the eggs in a small pot filled with enough water to cover them. Bring to the boil over a high heat. Remove from the heat, cover with a lid, and let them sit for 10 minutes. Drain the water, and set the eggs in a bowl of cold water to stop the cooking process. I find they're easier to peel when made a day or two in advance.

Pork Fried Cauliflower Couscous

Serves 2

This is a great way to use up extra Cauliflower Couscous (page 139). In fact, it's a great reason to make the Cauliflower Couscous so you can reap the rewards of leftovers—just be sure to make it at least a day in advance since it needs to be cold to work best in this dish.

Calories	342
Fat	29.5
Protein	16.6
Carbs	5.8
Fiber	1.1
Net carbs	4.7

1 tablespoon olive oil

2 eggs, beaten

Sea salt & freshly ground black pepper

2 boneless pork chops, diced

1 tablespoon sesame oil

1 teaspoon freshly grated ginger

1 garlic clove, chopped fine

3 cups leftover Cauliflower Couscous

3 tablespoons soy sauce

2 to 3 spring onions, chopped

Heat 1 teaspoon of olive oil in a deep frying pan over a medium-high heat until shimmering. Add the eggs, season with salt and pepper and cook, stirring, until cooked through, about 1 minute. Transfer to a small bowl.

Increase the heat to high, and add the rest of olive oil to the pan. Add the pork, and sauté until golden and cooked through, 2 to 3 minutes. Transfer to the bowl with the eggs.

Heat the sesame oil in the same skillet. Add the ginger and garlic. Sauté until fragrant, 15 to 30 seconds. Add the cauliflower couscous, making sure to break up any clumps. Stir in the soy sauce and spring onions. Add the pork and egg back to the pan. Sauté until the cauliflower couscous is heated through, 1 to 2 minutes. Serve hot.

DINNER

Kimchi Pork Lettuce Cups

Thai Turkey Burger

BBQ Flank Steak & Cabbage Slaw

Beef Bolognese

Smoky Butter Roast Chicken

Chicken Fajita Bowls

Almond-crusted Salmon Patties

Swedish Meatballs

Magic Keto Pizza

Kimchi Pork Lettuce Cups

Serves 2

This Korean-inspired dish packs a punch of flavor. To eat, scoop up some of the pork filling with a lettuce leaf, roll up, and dig in. For a different twist, you can drop the lettuce, and serve the filling tossed with courgetti.

Calories	322
Fat	24.3
Protein	19.7
Carbs	6.8
Fiber	2.6
Net carbs	4.2

2 teaspoons extra virgin olive oil
1 garlic clove, chopped fine
8 ounces ground pork
Handful of fresh coriander, chopped
½ cup kimchi, chopped fine
1 teaspoon fish sauce (Red Boat fish sauce has no added sugar)
1½ teaspoons soy sauce
Sea salt, to taste
1 small head of Boston lettuce, leaves removed, rinsed & patted dry
Lime wedges, for garnish
Fresh mint, for garnish

In a 10-inch frying pan, heat the oil over a medium-high heat until shimmering. Add the garlic, and sauté until lightly golden, 1 to 2 minutes. Add the pork, using a fork to break up any large chunks. Add the coriander, kimchi, fish sauce, and soy sauce. Season with salt. Reduce heat to medium-low. Continue cooking, stirring every couple of minutes, until the pork is completely cooked through, 7 to 9 minutes.

Meanwhile, arrange the lettuce leaves on a platter.

Spoon the cooked pork filling over the lettuce leaves. Garnish with lime wedges and fresh mint. Serve immediately.

Thai Turkey Burger

Serves 2

These burgers pack a punch of flavor, in all the good ways. If you've got some carbs to spare, and are really craving a bun for them, make the Easy Keto Bread on page 129 to serve them on. The Courgette Fries on page 142 are a must!

Calories	451
Fat	29
Protein	45.5
Carbs	1.8
Fiber	0.8
Net carbs	1

12 ounces ground turkey
1 garlic clove, chopped fine
1 teaspoon fresh grated ginger
Handful of fresh coriander, stems & leaves chopped fine
2 teaspoons red curry paste
½ teaspoon sea salt, plus more to taste
4 teaspoons mayonnaise
½ teaspoon Dijon mustard
Freshly ground black pepper
2 teaspoons extra virgin olive oil
2 romaine heart leaves or curly kale leaves

In a medium bowl, add the turkey, garlic, ginger, half of the chopped coriander, curry paste, and salt. Mix well. Divide the mixture into 2 equal portions, and shape into flat 4-inch patties.

In a small bowl, mix together the mayonnaise, Dijon, and remaining coriander. Season with salt and pepper.

Heat the oil in a frying pan over medium-high heat. Add the burgers, and cook until browned underneath, 4 to 5 minutes. Flip, and continue cooking until browned on other side, and cooked through, 4 to 5 minutes more.

Wrap each burger in a lettuce leaf to serve.

BBQ Flank Steak & Cabbage Slaw

Serves 4

The butter sounds like an odd addition to BBQ sauce, but it creates a thick, rich sauce and adds extra fat to a particularly lean cut of meat.

Calories	392
Fat	25
Protein	37
Carbs	3
Fiber	1
Net carbs	2

¼ cup ketchup (a no added sugar variety like Primal Kitchen)
2 tablespoons butter, melted
1 teaspoon Dijon mustard
½ teaspoon onion powder
½ teaspoon Worcestershire sauce
½ teaspoon freshly ground black pepper, plus more as needed
1½ pound flank steak
¼ cup mayonnaise
1 tablespoon apple cider vinegar
¼ teaspoon celery seed
Sea salt, to taste
2 cups shredded cabbage

Preheat the grill in your oven to high with the rack positioned under the grill.

In a small bowl, whisk together the ketchup, butter, mustard, onion powder, Worcestershire sauce, and black pepper.

Place the steak on a rimmed sheet pan. Brush the sauce all over, top and bottom. Cook 5 to 7 minutes, until nicely browned on top. Turn, and cook 5 to 7 minutes more, to desired doneness. Let rest for 5 minutes.

Meanwhile, prepare the slaw. In a small bowl, whisk together the mayonnaise, vinegar, and celery seed in a deep bowl. Season with salt and pepper. Add the cabbage, and stir until well mixed. Set aside in the fridge. This may be prepared 1 day in advance.

Slice the steak, cutting against the grain, and serve with the slaw.

Note: If you're planning ahead, you can marinate the steak 1 to 2 days in advance by placing it in a ziptop bag with the sauce in the fridge. Cook as directed.

Beef Bolognese

Serves 4

Pasta is one thing many miss when first starting Keto. Here the sauce gets all the attention, which you'll see is for good reason once you taste a spoonful. It's perfect served over courgetti, but you can also go for an Italian sloppy Joe, and serve it on Easy Keto Bread (page 129).

Calories	532
Fat	36.2
Protein	42.6
Carbs	8.4
Fiber	3.7
Net carbs	3.7

4 slices thick-cut bacon, chopped
1½ pounds ground beef
Sea salt & freshly ground black pepper
¾ cup double cream
1 (28-ounce) can tomato puree
Courgetti, to serve (page 141)
Grated Parmesan cheese, to serve (optional)

Add the bacon to a cold deep frying pan, and place over medium-high heat. Cook until crisp all over, turning once. Transfer to a bowl using a slotted spoon.

Crumble the beef into the skillet. Season with salt and pepper. Cook, stirring occasionally, until well browned, 5 to 7 minutes.

Reduce the heat to medium-low. Stir in the cream. Cook, stirring occasionally, until any liquid has mostly evaporated, but the meat isn't dry, about 10 minutes.

Stir in the tomato puree, making sure to scrape up any browned bits from the bottom of the pan. Season with salt. Bring to the boil. Reduce heat to low. Cook for 2 to 3 hours, stirring occasionally. Add a few tablespoons of water, as needed, to prevent the sauce from sticking to the pan.

About 30 minutes before the sauce is ready, begin preparing the Courgetti on page 141.

Serve the bolognese over the courgetti, with Parmesan, if desired.

Note: Once you add the tomato puree to the pan, you can transfer the sauce to a slow cooker, and cook on low for 4 to 6 hours.

Smoky Butter Roast Chicken

Serves 4

Two things to know when making the perfect roast chicken: high heat is your friend, and you don't need to truss it (tie the legs and wings back). Sure, trussing looks pretty, but leaving the chicken as-is allows the heat to circulate, helping it cook faster and evenly. For a simpler version of this recipe, omit the paprika, garlic and herbs from the butter.

Calories	614
Fat	51
Protein	37
Carbs	0.5
Fiber	0
Net carbs	0.5

6 tablespoons butter, softened
1½ teaspoons smoked paprika
1 garlic clove, grated
Handful of fresh flat-leaf parsley, chopped
Sea salt and freshly ground black pepper, to taste
1 (3½ pound) whole chicken

Preheat the oven to 450°F (230°C).

In a small bowl, combine the butter, paprika, garlic, parsley, salt and pepper. Using a fork, mix together until well blended.

Place the chicken in a roasting pan. Rub the butter mixture all over. Cook for 20 minutes, then add ½ cup of water to the bottom of the pan—this helps prevent the drippings from smoking, while making a natural sauce with the juices. Roast for 40 to 50 minutes more, basting every 15 minutes, until the juices run clear and an instant-read thermometer inserted in the thigh registers 165°F (75°C).

Remove the chicken from the oven and let sit for 5 to 10 minutes before carving.

Chicken Fajita Bowls

Serves 2

Who can resist this flavoursome Tex-Mex dish? Perfect when served with Cauliflower Couscous for a satisfying, spicy supper.

Calories	455
Fat	32
Protein	36.3
Carbs	6
Fiber	2.3
Net carbs	3.7

2 chicken thighs, skin-on
2 chicken legs, skin-on
2 to 3 tablespoons butter, softened
1 teaspoon taco seasoning (be sure to choose one without hidden sweeteners)
Sea salt and freshly ground black pepper
1 poblano pepper, seeded and sliced
2 garlic cloves, chopped
1 tablespoon extra virgin olive oil
Cauliflower Couscous (page 139)
1 lime, zested then cut into quarters
Small bunch of fresh coriander, leaves and stems chopped

Preheat the oven to 450°F (230°C).

Rub the chicken pieces all over with butter. Place in a single layer in a 9-inch by 13-inch roasting pan. Sprinkle with the taco spice; season with salt and pepper. Add the poblano and garlic to the pan, and drizzle with the olive oil.

Roast until the chicken begins to brown, 15 to 20 minutes. Give the peppers a stir to coat with the pan juices. Add a few tablespoons of water if the pan seems too dry. Spoon some of the juices over the chicken. Bake for 15 to 20 minutes more, until the chicken reaches 165°F when tested with an instant-read thermometer.

Meanwhile, prepare the cauliflower couscous as directed on page 139. Once cooked, stir in the lime zest and half the coriander.

To serve, divide the couscous between two wide, shallow bowls. Top each with a chicken leg and thigh, and some of the peppers. Spoon the pan juices on top. Sprinkle with the remaining coriander, and enjoy!

Almond-Crusted Salmon Patties

Serves 4

Some people notice an uptick in their grocery bills when switching to Keto. Using canned salmon gives you more bang for your buck, while you're still getting the benefits of Omega-3 plus a boost of calcium.

Calories	369
Fat	26
Protein	26
Carbs	7
Fiber	3.5
Net carbs	3.5

2 (6-ounce) cans wild pink salmon
1 tablespoon Dijon mustard
¼ teaspoon paprika
Handful of fresh flat-leaf parsley, chopped
1 large egg
Sea salt and freshly ground black pepper, to taste
1 cup almond meal
2 tablespoons coconut oil

In the bowl of a food processor, combine the salmon, mustard, paprika, parsley, egg, salt, pepper, and ½ a cup of the almond meal. Pulse until the mixture is coarsely blended (a few chunks of salmon still remaining). Transfer to a bowl, cover, and chill in the fridge for at least 1 hour, or overnight.

When ready to cook, divide the salmon mixture into 8 even balls. Flatten then into patties. Use the remaining ½ cup of almond meal to coat them all over.

In a 10-inch nonstick frying pan, melt 1 tablespoon of coconut oil over a medium heat until shimmering. Add the patties to the pan (you may need to do this in batches, so as to not overcrowd the pan). Cook until golden underneath, 3 to 4 minutes. Turn, and cook until golden on the other side, 3 to 4 minutes more. Serve hot.

Swedish Meatballs

Serves 2

A Keto on the traditional Swedish favourite. Fun to make and delicious to eat.

Calories	728
Fat	2650.7
Protein	59.6
Carbs	8.4
Fiber	2.8
Net carbs	5.6

1 pound ground beef
1 egg
1 garlic clove, grated
¼ teaspoon fresh grated nutmeg
2 tablespoons chopped fresh flat-leaf parsley
¼ cup almond flour
½ teaspoon sea salt
Freshly ground black pepper, to taste
2 tablespoons butter
1 tablespoon Dijon mustard (be sure to buy one
    without added sugar)
1 teaspoon tamari
2 teaspoons coconut flour
¾ cup chicken or beef broth
½ cup double cream

In a medium bowl, add the beef, egg, garlic, nutmeg, parsley, almond flour, salt, and pepper. Stir together with your hands, or a wooden spoon if that's more comfortable, until well mixed. Shape into 8 balls.

Melt the butter in an 8-inch frying pan over a medium-high heat. Add the meatballs. Cook until browned all over, turning as needed, 8 to 10 minutes. Transfer to a dish; set aside.

Discard all but 1 tablespoon of the fat from the pan. Over a medium heat, stir in the mustard, tamari, and coconut flour, scraping up any browned bits. Stir in the broth. Bring to a boil. Reduce heat to a simmer, and stir in the cream. Season with salt and pepper. Add the meatballs back to the pan, and cook 8 to 10 minutes more, until the sauce thickens. Serve hot.

Magic Keto Pizza

Serves 2 to 4

Pizza is one food I hear lots of people miss when cutting out carbs. As an Italian girl from Brooklyn, I understand this very well, and am really excited to share this recipe. Let's be real, nothing will ever compare to a traditional crust, but this crust is truly amazing, and magical in its own right. The real test is holding up a slice that defies gravity, and doesn't flop over! The only thing you're left to ponder is to fold, or not fold, as you devour it.

Calories	169
Fat	10
Protein	16
Carbs	5.4
Fiber	2
Net carbs	3.4
Analysis per slice	

For the crust
1 egg
6 ounces shredded mozzarella cheese
4 tablespoons butter, softened and broken into chunks
½ cup superfine blanched almond flour
6 tablespoons coconut flour, plus extra for dusting
2 teaspoons baking powder
¼ teaspoon sea salt

For the pizza

¾ cup Slow-Simmered Tomato Sauce (page 132)

6 ounces mozzarella cheese, shredded

Any desired keto-friendly toppings

Preheat the oven to 375°F (190°C).

To make the crust, place the egg, mozzarella, butter, flours, baking powder and sea salt to the bowl of a food processor. Pulse until it forms a rough ball. Very lightly dust a counter with coconut flour. Knead the dough until it becomes smooth, 30 to 60 seconds, only adding more coconut flour as needed to keep the dough from sticking.

Place the dough on a sheet of parchment or waxed paper. Cover with another sheet. Roll into a ⅛-inch thick circle. Remove the top layer of parchment. Slide the crust, still on the parchment paper onto a pizza pan or a large baking sheet. Bake until lightly golden, about 15 minutes.

Spread the tomato sauce on top, leaving a ¼ to ½-inch border at the edge. Sprinkle with mozzarella cheese and add any desired toppings. Bake until the cheese is melted and bubbling, and the crust is crispy, 15 to 20 minutes more. Let rest for 2 minutes before slicing and serving.

To heat leftovers, add the slices to a nonstick pan over medium heat. Cook until hot and enjoy.

TREATS & BEVERAGES

Orange Espresso Chia Pudding

Chocolate Almond Butter Cup Fat Bombs

Almond Joy Avocado Mousse

Berry Cheesecake Bars

Coconut Whipped Cream

Mocha Bulletproof Coffee

Bulletproof Coconut Chai

Orange Espresso Chia Pudding

Serves 2

I'm convinced there's a chia pudding conspiracy out there. Every recipe you read directs you to chill them overnight—I've never had success with this method, as chia seeds really need a full 24 hours to properly absorb the liquid and plump up. So, plan ahead when making these. The good news is the recipe can be doubled, and they keep for a few days in the fridge, so you can make a batch if you like, and enjoy chia pudding all week long.

Note: Oranges aren't allowed on Keto but you can use the zest with abandon since all the sugar is in the fruit itself.

Calories	206
Fat	14.4
Protein	7.2
Carbs	14.9
Fiber	10.1
Net carbs	4.8

¾ cup unsweetened almond milk
2 tablespoons espresso or strongly brewed coffee
Zest of 1 orange
1 packet stevia powder (optional)
4 tablespoons white chia seeds
2 tablespoons sliced almonds, toasted

In a small bowl, whisk together the almond milk, espresso, orange zest, and stevia, if using. Stir in the chia seeds until well mixed.

Divide between two 8-ounce mason jars. Cover with the lid. Chill for at least 24 hours. The pudding will keep, covered, for up to **4 days**. To serve, top each pudding with half the almonds.

Chocolate Almond Butter Cup Fat Bombs

Makes 12

What other diet will allow you to eat anything as sinful-tasting as this? You might have to hide them from the kids!

Calories	135
Fat	13.4
Protein	2.2
Carbs	6
Fiber	2.8
Net carbs	3.2

6 tablespoons dark chocolate chips (Lily's are sweet-
    ened with stevia)
6 tablespoons almond butter
6 tablespoons coconut oil
1 packet stevia powder

Line a 12-cup mini muffin tin with paper liners.

In a small microwave-safe bowl, melt the chocolate chips in 30-second intervals. Pour half into the prepared tin cups. Let cool for 5 minutes.

In a small pan, combine the almond butter and coconut oil over a low heat. Cook until melted, stirring together to mix. Stir in the stevia. Pour an even amount over the chocolate in the paper liners.

Evenly pour the remaining chocolate over the almond butter filling. Set in the fridge to firm up, at least 2 hours. Keep refrigerated.

Almond Joy Avocado Mousse

Serves 2

Avocado is a clever ingredient in this sumptuous sweet dish. The smooth, velvety texture is to die for.

Calories	268
Fat	37
Protein	263.4
Carbs	22.7
Fiber	13
Net carbs	9.7

1 ripe avocado, pitted and fruit scooped from skin
1 to 2 packets stevia powder
2 tablespoons cocoa powder
½ teaspoon vanilla extract
6 to 8 tablespoons coconut milk (depends on size of avocado)
1 tablespoon dark chocolate chips
1 tablespoon coconut flakes
1 tablespoon sliced almonds
Coconut Whipped Cream, to serve (optional, page 121)

Place the avocado, stevia, cocoa powder, vanilla, and coconut milk in the bowl of a food processor.

Pulse until smooth.

Evenly spoon the pudding into 2 small bowls or jars. Top evenly with the chocolate chips, coconut flakes, and almonds. Cover with clingfilm, and chill for at least 2 hours, until the pudding is set. It can be made up to 1 day in advance. Top with Coconut Whipped Cream before serving, if using.

Berry Cheesecake Bars

Makes 8 bars

Literally the perfect snack. Make these in advance and keep in your bag for those busy days when you are constantly on the move

Calories	229
Fat	21.7
Protein	5.6
Carbs	5.7
Fiber	1.6
Net carbs	4.1
Analysis based on one bar	

For the crust
3 tablespoons butter, melted
1 cup almond flour
1 packet stevia powder

For the filling
8 ounces full-fat cream cheese, softened
1 egg
2 packets stevia powder
1 teaspoon lemon juice
¼ cup raspberries or blueberries

Preheat the oven to 350°F (180°C).

Line an 8-inch loaf tin with a piece of parchment paper long enough to hang over the slides (this acts as a sling to lift the bars out when done).

To make the crust, combine the butter, almond flour, and stevia in a small bowl. Stir until mixed, then press into the bottom of the prepared tin. Bake until set, 7 to 8 minutes. Let cool completely.

To make the filling, combine the cream cheese, egg, stevia, and lemon juice in a medium bowl. Stir with a fork until well blended. Spoon over the crust.

Mash the berries lightly with the back of a fork, just to break them up a bit. Scatter over the filling, and use a butter knife to swirl them through the cream cheese mixture.

Bake for 15 to 20 minutes until the center is mostly set (it'll jiggle slightly like jelly). Let cool completely, then chill for at least 3 hours, or overnight, before cutting into 8 even bars.

Coconut Whipped Cream

Makes 1 cup (serving size one tablespoon)

Making a keto-friendly whipped cream at home is easier than you think! All it requires is advance planning, since the canned coconut milk needs to be chilled for a full day in order for it to whip properly. It's perfect for topping the Almond Joy Avocado Mousse on page 117, or just add some berries for a quick snack. Want to jazz it up? Try adding a dash of cinnamon, 1 teaspoon of cocoa, or some citrus zest before you whip it.

Calories	61
Fat	6.3
Protein	0.6
Carbs	1.4
Fiber	0.6
Net carbs	0.8

1 (15-ounce) can full-fat unsweetened coconut milk

Place the can of coconut milk in the fridge 24 hours before you plan to make this whipped cream.

The next day, open the can, scoop out the solids and add them to a small bowl (save the remaining coconut water for another use). Using a handheld mixer, whip the coconut solids until fluffy and thickened into a slightly stiff cream. Use immediately.

Mocha Bulletproof Coffee

Serves 1

When you need a quick boost of energy that also leaves you feeling full, bulletproof coffee is the way to go. The butter and MCT oil bulk it out into a satisfying mini meal. It's a great way to start the day, or as an afternoon pick-me-up to keep snacking at bay. Should you want a little sweet touch, you can add ½ a packet of stevia powder; anything more will accentuate coffee's natural bitter notes.

Calories	327
Fat	39.4
Protein	0.7
Carbs	0
Fiber	0
Net carbs	0

¾ cup hot brewed coffee
2 tablespoons butter
1 tablespoon MCT oil (optional)
½ teaspoon cocoa powder
¼ teaspoon cinnamon

Place all the ingredients in a blender bowl. Blend on high for 30 to 60 seconds until frothy.

Bulletproof Coconut Chai

Serves 1

Traditional chai is loaded with sugar. This version, a tea relative of the popular bulletproof coffee, delivers all the aromatic flavors, plus a boost of energy, without being cloyingly sweet.

Calories	464
Fat	51
Protein	3.5
Carbs	7
Fiber	1
Net carbs	6

12 ounces hot brewed black tea
2 tablespoons butter
1 tablespoon MCT oil
¼ cup unsweetened coconut milk
¼ teaspoon cardamom
¼ teaspoon fresh grated ginger
¼ teaspoon ground cloves
½ teaspoon cinnamon

Place all the ingredients in a blender bowl. Blend on high for 30 to 60 seconds until frothy.

BASICS

Slow-Roasted Chicken Bone Broth

Easy Keto Bread

Slow-Simmered Tomato Sauce

Homemade Ranch Dressing

Easy Homemade Vinaigrette

Homemade Parmesan Crisps

Cauliflower Couscous

Courgetti

Courgette Fries

Slow-Roasted Chicken Bone Broth

Makes about 1 litre

There is something intrinsically comforting about this soothing Chicken Bone Broth. Just like your grandmother would have made.

Calories	40
Fat	0.3
Protein	9.4
Carbs	0.6
Fiber	0
Net carbs	0.6
Analysis based on one cup	

8 chicken thighs, skin on and bone-in
3 garlic cloves, smashed
4 celery sticks, cut into 2-inch pieces
Sea salt and freshly ground black pepper
3 tablespoons extra virgin olive oil
Handful of fresh flat-leaf parsley

Preheat your oven to 475°F (240°C), with the rack adjusted to the upper center position.

Arrange the chicken pieces, garlic, and celery in a 9-inch by 13-inch roasting pan. Season with salt and pepper. Roast for 15 minutes.

Drizzle the oil on top. Roast for 15 more minutes.

Add the parsley, and pour 6 cups of water into the pan. Roast for 30 more minutes.

Reduce the oven temperature to 275°F (135°C). Roast for at least 3 hours, and up to 6 hours, adding more water to the pan as needed to keep the chicken covered by about two-thirds. You want the tops to get nicely browned but keep them mostly submerged so the meat braises. Taste the broth as it cooks, and add more salt, as needed.

Using a slotted spoon, transfer the chicken to a plate. Once cooled, remove the meat, and discard the bones. The chicken is perfect as a simple sandwich on Easy Keto Bread (page 129)—don't forget the mayo! It can also be used in the Cobb Salad on page 86 instead of Salmon, or the Chicken Caesar Salad on page 80.

Strain the stock, discarding any solids. Let the stock cool completely, then pack in containers, and refrigerate for up to 1 week, or store in the freezer for up to 2 months.

Easy Keto Bread

Serves 1 to 2

Yes, bread is really possibly on Keto. Hello, avocado toast! Unlike so many of the Keto bread recipes out there, this one doesn't taste eggy. I really love the microwave version, but I'm including an option to bake it, too. The baked version is lighter in texture, and must cool completely before using or it'll crumble. The microwave bread is PERFECT for slicing and toasting when you want bread in less than 2 minutes (no joke). The texture reminds me of crumpets with all the nooks and crannies, and is lovely toasted in a pan with some butter (a conventional toaster works, too).

Note: The smaller size is perfect for sliders, while the larger makes a great burger bun.

Calories	194
Fat	18
Protein	5.5
Carbs	4.5
Fiber	2
Net carbs	2.5

2 tablespoons butter, melted

1 large egg

1 tablespoon water or almond milk

2 tablespoons almond flour

1 tablespoon coconut flour

½ teaspoon baking powder

⅛ teaspoon sea salt

Microwave Method:

Use a pastry brush to coat the sides and bottoms of two 3½-inch (6 ounce) or one 5-inch (10 ounce) microwave-safe ramekin with some of the butter.

In a small bowl, whisk together the egg and water or almond milk. Whisk in the flours, baking powder, and salt.

Scrape the batter into the prepared ramekin or ramekins. Cook on high for 60 to 90 seconds for small breads and 1 to 2 minutes for larger ones, until cooked through (cook small ramekins one at a time for best results). Test for doneness by gently tapping the center with your finger, and if it springs back that means it's cooked through. Let cool for 1 minute. Slide a knife around the inside rim to loosen the bread. Turn out onto a board. Slice in half, and use as you would sandwich bread.

Oven Method:

Preheat the oven to 400°F (200°C). Cut out parchment circles to line the bottom of two 3½-inch (6 ounce) or one 5-inch (10 ounce) oven-safe ramekin. Generously grease the sides with butter.

In a small bowl, whisk together the egg and water or almond milk. Whisk in the flours, baking powder, and salt.

Scrape the batter into the prepared ramekin or ramekins. Bake for 12 to 18 minutes until cooked through; start checking smaller ones at 10 minutes (a skewer inserted in the center should come out clean—don't test too soon or you'll deflate the bread). Let cool completely, then slice in half, and use as you would sandwich bread.

Slow-Simmered Tomato Sauce

Makes about 3½ cups

You can make this incredibly versatile sauce in bulk and freeze in batches.

Calories	88
Fat	8.3
Protein	1
Carbs	4.3
Fiber	2.2
Net carbs	2.1
Analysis based on ½ cup	

1 (28-ounce) can San Marzano Tomatoes,
    whole and peeled
3 garlic cloves, smashed
¼ cup extra virgin olive oil
½ teaspoon dried basil
Sea salt, to taste

Place the tomatoes in a blender, and puree until smooth. You can alternatively just crush them with your hands into the pan if you prefer a chunkier-style sauce.

Add the tomatoes, garlic, olive oil, basil, and salt to a deep frying pan. Cook, *uncovered*, for 45 minutes over a low heat. Around 15 to 20 minutes into the cooking time, it'll start simmering vigorously—don't worry, that's what it should be doing.

After 45 minutes, the sauce is ready to serve, or you can transfer it to a jar, let cool completely, and store in the fridge for up 3 days, or the freezer for up to 2 months.

Homemade Ranch Dressing

Makes 1 cup (serving size one tablespoon)

Quick and easy – this sauce adds a zing to any meat dish.

Calories	60
Fat	6.2
Protein	0.6
Carbs	0.6
Fiber	0
Net carbs	0.6

½ cup mayonnaise
½ cup sour cream
2 teaspoons freshly squeezed lemon juice
1 teaspoon apple cider vinegar
Handful of fresh chives, chopped
Sea salt and freshly ground black pepper

Whisk the mayonnaise, sour cream, lemon juice, and vinegar with 2 tablespoons water in a medium bowl. Stir in the chives. Season with salt and pepper. Pour ino a jar and refrigerate for up to 1 week. **Shake well** before each use.

Easy Homemade Vinaigrette

Makes ¾ cup (serving size one tablespoon)

It happens, we all get busy, and some mornings it's impossible to pack lunch. Keep a stash of this homemade dressing in your desk drawer, and you can always pull a keto-friendly lunch together from the salad bar. Stick to plain items, raw or steamed to ensure there's no hidden sweeteners, and grab a few hard boiled eggs to bulk it out with extra fat and protein. Don't worry about the herbs spoiling at room temperature—there's enough vinegar in the dressing to preserve them.

Calories	83
Fat	9.5
Protein	0.1
Carbs	0.1
Fiber	0
Net carbs	0.1

½ cup extra virgin olive oil
¼ cup red wine vinegar
2 teaspoons wholegrain mustard
Chopped fresh herbs of your choice (chives, coriander, parsley, spring onions)
Sea salt and freshly ground black pepper, to taste

Place all of the ingredients in a mason jar. Cover tightly. Shake until well blended. Will keep at room temperature for up to 1 month. Be sure to shake well before each use.

Homemade Parmesan Crisps

Makes 12

Get your crisp fix with these easy-to-make cheese versions. All you need is one ingredient and less than 10 minutes. They double as amazing croutons in salad (see the Chicken Caesar Salad with Parmesan Crisps on page 80).

Calories	38
Fat	2.5
Protein	3.5
Carbs	0.3
Fiber	0
Net carbs	0.3

2 ounces Pecorino cheese, finely grated

Oven Method:
Preheat the oven to 350°F (180°C). Line a baking sheet with a silicon mat or parchment paper.

Drop the cheese into 12 mounds (about 2 tablespoons each) onto the sheet, leaving 1 inch between so they have room to spread.

Bake for 5 to 7 minutes until golden and bubbly. They'll be soft when they come out of the oven, but will crisp up within a few minutes of cooling.

Stove-top Method:

Heat a nonstick pan over a medium-low heat. Drop mounds of cheese into the pan (about 2 tablespoons each). Cook until the cheese melts and gets golden around the edges, about 2 minutes. Use an offset spatula to loosen and flip them. Cook 1 to 2 minutes more. Transfer to a plate and let cool for a few minutes to crisp up.

Cauliflower Couscous

Serves 2

One taste, and you'll wonder where this simple side has been your whole life. The key is to stir the cauliflower couscous constantly while it cooks to help the water evaporate as it releases from the cauliflower, otherwise it might steam and get mushy. A delicious variation is Cauliflower Couscous with lime and coriander on page 139.

Calories	116
Fat	11.8
Protein	1.3
Carbs	2.6
Fiber	1.4
Net carbs	1.2

Small head of cauliflower, florets only (save stems for another use)
2 tablespoons butter
Sea salt and freshly ground pepper, to taste

Place the florets in a food processor. Pulse until broken down into fine bits resembling couscous.

In a deep nonstick pan, melt 1 tablespoon of butter.

Add the cauliflower, cook until tender, stirring constantly, 5 to 7 minutes. Stir in the remaining tablespoon of butter. Season with salt and pepper. Fluff with a fork before serving.

Courgetti

Serves 2

It might seem silly to have a recipe for courgetti alone but there's more to making it than just spiralizing courgettes.

Calories	107
Fat	11.6
Protein	0.8
Carbs	0.8
Fiber	0.3
Net carbs	0.5

3 medium courgettes
2 tablespoons butter
Sea salt, to taste
Special equipment: spiralizer

Spiralize the courgettes into thin noodles. Lay a clean kitchen towel on the counter. Spread the noodles on the towel, and sprinkle with a little salt. This helps draw out excess water. Pat the noodles dry.

In a deep frying pan, melt the butter over a medium heat. Add the courgetti. Saute for 1 minute. You want them to stay a little raw to retain their texture. Then they're ready to eat, serve as a side, or use in another dish, like the Spicy Sesame Courgetti (page 74).

Courgette Fries

Serves 2

Thanks to low-carb courgettes you don't have to say goodbye to fries!

Calories	120
Fat	8
Protein	10.9
Carbs	1.1
Fiber	0.1
Net carbs	1

1 medium courgette
1 egg, beaten
½ cup finely grated Parmesan cheese

Preheat the oven to 425°F (220°C) with the rack in the lowest position. Line a rimmed baking sheet with parchment paper.

Trim the courgette ends. Cut the courgettes in half lengthways, then cut each half into ¼-inch thick strips. Dip each piece of courgette into the egg, shaking off any excess, then toss in the cheese. Arrange the coated courgettes in a single layer on the prepared baking sheet.

Bake for 25 to 30 minutes, turning halfway through, until crisp and golden. Serve hot.

Part III

Resources

Measurement Conversion Chart

DRY measurements

1 cup	= 16 tbsp	= 48 tsp	= 250 ml
¾ cup	= 12 tbsp	= 36 tsp	= 175 ml
⅔ cup	= 10⅔ tbsp	= 32 tsp	= 150 ml
⅓ cup	= 8 tbsp	= 24 tsp	= 125 ml
½ cup	= 5⅓ tbsp	= 16 tsp	= 75 ml
¼ cup	= 4 tbsp	= 12 tsp	= 50 ml
⅛ cup	= 2 tbsp	= 6 tsp	= 30 ml
⅟₁₆ cup	= 1 tbsp	= 3 tsp	= 15 ml

LIQUID measurements

1 gal	= 4 qt	= 16 cup	= 128 fl oz
½ gal	= 2 qt	= 8 cup	= 64 fl oz
¼ gal	= 1 qt	= 4 cup	= 32 fl oz
⅛ gal	= ½ qt	= 2 cup	= 16 fl oz
⅟₁₆ gal	= ¼ qt	= 1 cup	= 8 fl oz

Meal Planner 1: Meals noon to 6pm only

Use the following pages to plan what you are going to eat over the next 4 weeks!

Day 1

Morning	KETO
Noon	KETO
Before 6pm	KETO

Day 2

Morning	KETO
Noon	KETO
Before 6pm	KETO

Day 3

Morning	KETO	
Noon	KETO	
Before 6pm	KETO	

Day 4

Morning	KETO	
Noon	KETO	
Before 6pm	KETO	

Day 5

Morning	KETO
Noon	KETO
Before 6pm	KETO

Day 6

Morning	FAST
Noon	KETO
Before 6pm	KETO

Day 7

Morning	FAST
Noon	KETO
Before 6pm	KETO

Day 8

Morning	FAST
Noon	KETO
Midday Snack	KETO
Before 6pm	KETO

Day 9

Morning	FAST
Noon	KETO
Midday Snack	KETO
Before 6pm	KETO

Day 10

Morning	FAST
Noon	KETO
Midday Snack	KETO
Before 6pm	KETO

Day 11

Morning	FAST
Noon	KETO
Midday Snack	KETO
Before 6pm	KETO

Day 12

Morning	FAST
Noon	KETO
Midday Snack	KETO
Before 6pm	KETO

Day 13

Morning	FAST
Noon	KETO
Midday Snack	KETO
Before 6pm	KETO

Day 14

Morning	KETO
Noon	KETO
Midday Snack	None
Before 6pm	KETO

Day 15

Morning	FAST
Noon	KETO
Midday Snack	KETO
Before 6pm	KETO

Day 16

Morning	FAST
Noon	KETO
Midday Snack	KETO
Before 6pm	KETO

Day 17

Morning	FAST
Noon	KETO
Midday Snack	KETO
Before 6pm	KETO

Day 18

Morning	FAST
Noon	KETO
Midday Snack	KETO
Before 6pm	KETO

Day 19

Morning	FAST
Noon	KETO
Midday Snack	KETO
Before 6pm	KETO

Day 20

Morning	FAST
Noon	KETO
Midday Snack	KETO
Before 6pm	KETO

Day 21

Morning	KETO
Noon	KETO
Midday Snack	None
Before 6pm	KETO

Day 22

Morning	FAST
Noon	KETO
Midday Snack	KETO
Before 6pm	KETO

Day 23

Morning	FAST
Noon	KETO
Midday Snack	KETO
Before 6pm	KETO

Day 24

Morning	FAST
Noon	KETO
Midday Snack	KETO
Before 6pm	KETO

Day 25

Morning	FAST
Noon	KETO
Midday Snack	KETO
Before 6pm	KETO

Day 26

Morning	FAST
Noon	KETO
Midday Snack	KETO
Before 6pm	KETO

Day 27

Morning	FAST
Noon	KETO
Midday Snack	KETO
Before 6pm	KETO

Day 28

Morning	KETO
Noon	KETO
Midday Snack	None
Before 6pm	KETO

Meal Planner 2: Alternate Intermittent Fasting

Day 1

Morning	KETO
Noon	KETO
Before 6pm	KETO

Day 2

Morning	KETO
Noon	KETO
Before 6pm	KETO

Day 3

Morning	KETO
Noon	KETO
Before 6pm	KETO

Day 4

Morning	KETO
Noon	KETO
Before 6pm	KETO

Day 5

Morning	KETO
Noon	KETO
Before 6pm	KETO

Day 6

Morning	FAST
Noon	KETO
Before 6pm	KETO

Day 7

Morning	KETO
Noon	KETO
Before 6pm	FAST

Day 8

Morning	KETO
Noon	KETO
Before 6pm	FAST

Day 9

Morning	KETO
Noon	KETO
Before 6pm	FAST

Day 10

Morning	FAST
Noon	KETO
Before 6pm	KETO

Day 11

Morning	KETO
Noon	KETO
Before 6pm	FAST

Day 12

Morning	FAST
Noon	KETO
Before 6pm	KETO

Day 13

Morning	KETO
Noon	KETO
Before 6pm	KETO

Day 14

Morning	KETO
Noon	KETO
Before 6pm	FAST

Day 15

Morning	FAST
Noon	KETO
Before 6pm	KETO

Day 16

Morning	KETO
Noon	KETO
Before 6pm	FAST

Day 17

Morning	FAST
Noon	KETO
Before 6pm	KETO

Day 18

Morning	KETO
Noon	KETO
Before 6pm	FAST

Day 19

Morning	FAST
Noon	KETO
Before 6pm	KETO

Day 20

Morning	KETO
Noon	KETO
Before 6pm	KETO

Day 21

Morning	KETO
Noon	KETO
Before 6pm	FAST

Day 22

Morning	FAST
Noon	KETO
Before 6pm	KETO

Day 23

Morning	KETO
Noon	KETO
Before 6pm	FAST

Day 24

Morning	FAST
Noon	KETO
Before 6pm	KETO

Day 25

Morning	KETO
Noon	KETO
Before 6pm	FAST

Day 26

Morning	FAST
Noon	KETO
Before 6pm	KETO

Day 27

Morning	KETO
Noon	KETO
Before 6pm	KETO

Day 28

Morning	KETO
Noon	KETO
Before 6pm	FAST